THE VEGAN SOURCEBOOK

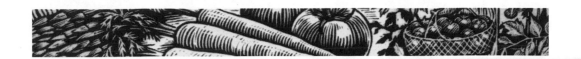

THE VEGAN SOURCEBOOK

SECOND EDITION

BY

JOANNE STEPANIAK, M.S.ED.

SPECIAL NUTRITION SECTION BY
VIRGINIA MESSINA, M.P.H., R.D.

FOREWORD BY CAROL J. ADAMS

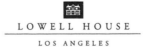

LOWELL HOUSE

LOS ANGELES

NTC/Contemporary Publishing Group

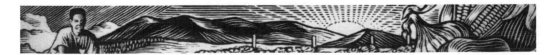

Library of Congress Cataloging in Publication Data

Stepaniak, Joanne, 1954–
    The vegan sourcebook / by Joanne Stepaniak ; special nutrition section by Virginia
Messina ; foreword by Carol J. Adams.—2nd ed.
      p. cm.
    Includes bibliographical references and index.
    ISBN 0-7373-0506-1 (pbk.)
     1. Veganism, 2. Vegan Cookery. I. Messina, Virginia. II. Title.

TX392.S73 2000
641.5'636—dc21

                                                 00-058634
                                                    CIP

Published by Lowell House, a division of NTC/Contemporary Publishing Group, Inc.
4255 West Touhy Avenue, Lincolnwood, Illinois 60646-1975, U.S.A.

Design by Laurie Young

Printed and bound in the United States of America
International Standard Book Number: 0-7373-0506-1
00 01 02 03 04 ML 18 17 16 15 14 13 12 11 10 9 8 7 6 5 4 3 2 1

To the animals:
May we be forgiven.

To the people:
May we learn to practice that which we most desire—
unconditional love.

PRAYER

We shall pass through this world but once.
Therefore, any good thing I can do,
For any living being,
Let me do it now.
Let me not defer it or neglect it,
For I shall not pass this way again.

—ANONYMOUS

Living Graves

We are the living graves of murdered beasts
Slaughtered to satisfy our appetites
We never pause to wonder at our feasts
If kine, like men, can possibly have rights
We pray on Sundays that we might have light
To guide our footsteps on the path we tread
We're sick of war—we do not want to fight—
The thought of it now fills our heart with dread.
And yet—we gorge ourselves upon the dead!
Like carrion crows we live and feed on meat,
Regardless of the suffering and pain
We cause by doing so. If thus we treat
Defenseless animals for sport or gain,
How can we hope in this world to attain
The peace we say we are so anxious for?

—George Bernard Shaw, 1856–1950

CONTENTS

FOREWORD

Joanne Stepaniak has been in my kitchen for years. Actually, her *cookbooks* have been in my kitchen for years. I have been a longtime admirer of her work. When it comes to recipes, I know that I can trust her. She has figured out how to balance seasonings, just how thick a soup should be, where and when to add nutritional yeast, and the myriad ways to incorporate tofu into a diet.

Perhaps that is why, when I received this book, I turned first to the recipes to learn what she had been thinking recently about food. I discovered in her tofu-vegetable spread a wonderful comfort food and a great food to share with nonvegans. But when we finish eating the wonderful tofu spread, will the compassion that motivated our choice of tofu also inform our interactions? In the pages that follow, Joanne Stepaniak tells us how and why it should.

Until I read *The Vegan Sourcebook*, I did not know that Joanne Stepaniak was such a wise person. Recipe books do not always convey an author's insights into what it means to be human and humane. But this book remedies that problem. Now, in one book, we can find the vegan perspective explained thoroughly and clearly.

Joanne's recipe book *Vegan Vittles* may have hinted at the depth and breadth of her approach to veganism. Specifically, she altered folk proverbs that drew upon outdated assumptions about our relationships to animals. Instead of "don't look a gift horse in the mouth," she proposed "don't look for bugs in a flower bouquet." For "don't put the cart before the horse," she suggested "don't slice the bread before it's baked." And instead of "talk turkey," she suggested "speak vegan."

Those were the clues that Joanne Stepaniak is not only creating recipes as she works in the kitchen. She benefits from what vegan cooking at its best does—gives us an opportunity to reflect on why we are preparing food in this way, with this care. We are not just mixing tofu and carrots and scallions to get the tofu spread, we are mixing our compassion for the world. With *The Vegan Sourcebook,* Joanne Stepaniak "speaks vegan" and we are in her debt for her clarity in crystallizing just how it is that veganism is compassion in action.

If you are new to veganism, you will find in these pages a cogent, intelligent, and insightful explanation of the history and ethics of veganism, and how to apply veganism to your own life. You will learn about the challenges and the rewards of veganism. In so many different ways, this book affirms that as you begin on this path, you are not alone. You are not alone in contemplating how our actions affect the suffering of animals, humans, and the earth—not alone in deciding to do something about this suffering. In becoming vegan, we need to see ourselves as part of a supportive network of like-minded people. This book makes that recognition possible. We meet like-minded people—Zoe, Michael, Tom, and others—who speak to us about their lives and their veganism, encouraging us wherever we are on the path.

If you are an experienced vegan, there is much for you as well. Joanne's discussion of the reasons for veganism helps us to recognize the human exploitation that accompanies animal agribusiness. By including a discussion of this, as well as of environmental racism, Joanne reminds us that the costs to people are also rightly our concern as vegans. Of equal importance is her discussion of our responsibilities, as vegans, to ourselves. The vegan ethic,

Joanne insists, includes taking care of our own "physical, mental, social, and emotional" needs. She convincingly tells us: "If the vegan ethic compels one to cherish and revere all life, one must certainly include oneself. Not to do so is to violate vegan precepts."

Just as she has brought us, joyfully, into new territory with her recipes, Joanne pulls us into an idea of veganism that resonates with all that is best in us: our caring about others, our sense of connectedness, our desire not to do harm. She describes how veganism changes us, deepening us, awakening us to new possibilities for ourselves. Joanne captures the transformational nature of veganism, drawing on the comments of vegans from diverse areas of life. She addresses issues such as anger—who doesn't feel that?—and how we should respond to animal abusers. She prepares us for the different stages of psychological adjustment to veganism.

Joanne illustrates how veganism leads us to be concerned about every form of animal exploitation, including circuses, zoos, hunting, rodeos, marine captivity parks, vivisection, horse and dog racing, xenotransplants, leather and wool productions, honey, companion animals, organic gardening, cosmetics, and hidden animal byproducts. She gracefully draws these diverse forms of harm to animals together into one ethic. Through her explanation, we can see how compassion intersects with so many aspects of our world.

I appreciate the sourcebook aspects of this book. I invite you to enjoy this wealth of material, from a description of hidden animal products to information on plant milks, from the Vegan Food Pyramid to vegan-friendly mail-order companies, from the scoop on why kosher foods may not be vegan to honey replacements. This material is here to make your veganism simpler.

An important contribution is the new definition of veganism Joanne provides. I agree with her that we should have a definition that is "prescriptive instead of prohibitive," that defines vegans by what we believe and are doing rather than by what we do not do. I am grateful to Joanne for this work in helping us recreate the vegan ethic to reflect our positive expression of connectedess.

Joanne describes how she went about augmenting her definition of veganism. The care with which she approached the issue enacts precisely what the definition conveys: "Veganism is an ethic that is committed to reverence and respect for all life and the planet that sustains it. Veganism brings with it the joy of living with peace of spirit and the comfort of knowing that one's thoughts, feelings, words, and actions have a strongly benevolent effect on the world." Joanne applied her definition of veganism to the very act of crafting this definition. Her model of "speaking vegan" is truly inspiring because she brings to this book the compassion that is its very subject. This is a model we can each embrace.

Why are you vegan? What do you eat? Here are the answers. And if you want to make your life simpler, make copies of Joanne's code of ethics (see pages 177–78) and hand them to people who inquire about your veganism. These two pages will make speaking vegan much easier.

These are some of the reasons I like *The Vegan Sourcebook*. I also appreciate the feelings it prompts as I read it. It is open, inviting, and informed. Its movement is always toward the positive, the affirmative. A negative proverb is rewritten to be positive; a definition that leans toward negation becomes one that affirms; a life that accepted suffering as inevitable becomes one that refuses to contribute to suffering. Joanne's voice throughout the book is one that tells us she wants the best for us, and helps us to want the best for ourselves, too.

—CAROL J. ADAMS, author of *The Sexual Politics of Meat: A Feminist-Vegetarian Critical Theory,* now in a tenth anniversary edition, and *The Inner Art of Vegetarianism: Spiritual Practices for Body and Soul*

PREFACE

For tens of thousands of years, humans coexisted peaceably and equitably with the other inhabitants of this planet. We used the gifts of nature that were within our reach, generally taking only what was necessary to survive. We left the world intact, much as we found it.

Only in the last few thousand years have humans so exploited the Earth—ravaged its bounty, unbalanced its cycles, poisoned its terrain, fouled its waters, polluted its air, and impeded the natural evolution of plants, insects, other animals, and ourselves. Perhaps it is a uniquely human trait to overconsume and desecrate our habitat; yet, as history proves, this has not always been our custom. What has made us so cynical, greedy, and hardened to the suffering and widespread disintegration of the natural world?

Somewhere along our journey we lost our way. Humans have become more and more segregated from those with whom we share the planet, making it easier to forget our place in the natural scheme of life. As we gain greater power to manipulate and destroy our environment, we alienate ourselves from it and view those who interfere with our "advancement" as enemies of progress. Despite our vast collection of material goods, nonindigenous Westernized humans have never felt more confused, stressed, violent, and isolated. We have become disenfranchised from the greater community of life, leaving us feeling at war with the natural elements and those who vie with us just to get their fair and rightful portion.

Western civilization focuses on the present and places great value on individual pleasure and enjoyment of the moment. Indigenous cultures more readily embrace a spirit of community and actively recognize that the present must be preserved for tomorrow. When we acknowledge the wisdom with which our ancestors lived, we may find the hope, courage, and guidance to change our current course of destruction.

There is little that separates humans from other sentient beings—we all feel pain, we all feel joy, we all deeply crave to be alive and to live freely, and we all share this planet together. The water, air, earth, and plants belong to no one except the community of life which connects us all.

If there is anything that differentiates humans from other living beings it may simply be the factor of choice. We have the option to heal or harm, nurture or destroy, respect or rape, protect or kill. The ability to choose does not necessarily elevate the human species, nor should one infer that it is a trait unique to humans. The capacity to choose should perhaps oblige us to be more responsible for our actions toward others. It is our duty to choose wisely, both collectively and individually, if we are ever again to find peace at any level.

Veganism advocates harmony, justice, and empathic living by acknowledging and respecting the interconnectedness of all life. It is an ethical beacon which can illuminate our moral path and steer us back toward reuniting with our global family. Its tenets can teach us how to live at peace with our world by becoming an integral part and defender of it.

This book details the broad principles and ethics that are the guideposts for people who practice a vegan lifestyle. Like many groups, the vegan community consists of men, women, and children of all ages and colors with diverse spiritual perspectives, cultural backgrounds, interests, and educational levels. The information contained herein is drawn from archives, conversations, and interviews with pioneers and participants at the forefront of the vegan movement, extensive research conducted by experts in their respective fields, as well as from my personal experience living as a vegan for over sixteen years and as a vegetarian for over thirty years. It is not intended to be the final word on vegan living, nor do I propose to be a spokesperson for all vegans. The topic of vegan living is complex and vast and destined for continued study by philosophers, ethicists, clergy, politicians, sociologists, educators, health-care practitioners, environmentalists, peace workers, animal advocates, and social activists. It is my sincere hope that by sharing information about veganism we can gain deeper understanding of what it means to be human and humane.

Joanne Stepaniak conducts compassionate living workshops and vegan cooking classes throughout North America. If you would like to arrange a presentation for your group of organization, please contact her at P.O. Box 82663, Swissvale, PA 15218, or visit her web site at www.vegsource.com/joanne.

Edict of Independence

Pity is the watchword
for unrecovered rebels
who never know the ecstasy
in conformity of self.
But I say joy is fleeting.
Perhaps it is the twisted mind
who sees with clarity
knots and gnarls and winding roads
that seduce the visionary,
horrify the sane.
I march to the rhythm of my own heart,
listening for footsteps gone or coming.
A breed united by differences.
Sick or sound?
Build an asylum to cage our souls,
choke our thoughts, smother our words.
We will rise again like ghouls from a crypt.
Truth knows no death.
Silence speaks no truth.
I sing our song of lunacy,
the heritage of heretics,
an anthem to the spirit
of those who have survived.

—JOANNE STEPANIAK, 1990

ACKNOWLEDGMENTS

The human spirit is not dead. It lives on in secret. . . . It has come to believe that compassion, in which all ethics must take root, can only attain its full breadth and depth if it embraces all living creatures and does not limit itself to mankind.

—ALBERT SCHWEITZER,
NOBEL PEACE PRIZE ADDRESS,
"THE PROBLEM OF PEACE
IN THE WORLD TODAY"

Special thanks to Bud Sperry, who had the insight to recognize the need for a book on vegan living and then endeavored to make it happen; to Maria Magallanes for her clarity, patience, and guidance in steering this project to completion; to Gene Bauston, an extraordinary person who has made great strides for veganism and had faith in my ability to bring such a project to fruition; to Michael Stepaniak, my best friend and lifemate, for his patience, guidance, endurance, insight, gentleness, commitment, and abiding love; to Michael Greger, for his acumen, sagacity, boundless energy, beautiful spirit, and heart of gold; to Ginny Messina, Norm Phelps, Brian Klocke, Mae Lee Sun, Freya Dinshah, Dean Smith, Stanley Sapon, Bret Davis, Syndee L'Ome Grace, and Ross Strader, who are among the kindest, most gifted, and most generous spirits I am privileged to know; and to Tom Regan, for his wisdom, inspiration, altruism, and infinite compassion. It is an honor to have the presence of all of you in this life and on these pages.

This book is a community venture in every sense. It would have been impossible without the contributions and support of numerous talented people who, when asked if they would be willing to assist, responded in the most vegan way possible—selflessly and magnanimously. Instead of being concerned about receiving individual credit for their efforts, they simply wanted to help get the message out about vegan living and the compassionate way of life. These are extremely busy, highly responsible individuals who donated time, research, wisdom, and knowledge so that others may fulfill their humane potential. Their generosity and collaborative energies demonstrate the true meaning of veganism. Each of these amazing people embodies the essence of love and compassion, which elevates the human spirit and makes the dream of a just world for all life imaginable.

The following people contributed expertise, research, writing, commentary, networking, access to vegan archives, editing, ideas, input, general assistance, support, and encouragement. They personify the vegan ethic in all that they do and symbolize the best of the human species. My gratitude to them is immeasurable:

Brian Barker, Gene Bauston, Will Bonsall, Andy Breslin, Elizabeth Conrey, Madge Darneille, Bret Davis, Karen Davis, Ph.D., Freya Dinshah, Jay Dinshah, Ann Cottrell Free, Brian Graff, Sharon Graff, Syndee L'Ome Grace, Michael Greger, M.D., Alex Hershaft, Ph.D., Brian Jacobs, Michael Klaper, M.D., Brian Klocke, Howard Lyman, Michael Markarian, Virginia Messina, M.P.H., R.D., Eric Mills, Hillary Morris, Marcia Pearson, Norm Phelps, Kevin Pickard, David Pimentel, Ph.D., Heidi Prescott, Tom Regan, Ph.D., Patti Rodgers, Julie Rosenfield, Stanley Sapon, Ph.D., Dean Smith, Michael Stepaniak, Ross Strader, Mae Lee Sun, Ethel Thurston, Molly Thorkildsen, Christina Vancheri, Donald Watson, Zoe Weil, Vernon Weir, and Brad Wolff.

Additional thanks to Peter Gilliver, chief general revision editor, and John Simpson of Oxford English Dictionaries in the United Kingdom.

Many people volunteered to be interviewed for this book in the hopes that their words and personal perspectives could provide support, guidance, encouragement, strength, and insight for those exploring the vegan path. They exposed their hearts so that others could grow. Mirrored in their benevolence is the soul of vegan living:

Lisa Robinson Bailey, Matt Ball, Gene Bauston, Rynn Berry, Jeffrey Brown, Sally Clinton, Jennie Collura, Amy Cottrill, Lorene Cox, Irene Cruikshank, Saurabh Dalal, Madge Darneille, Karen Davis, Ph.D., Freya Dinshah, Jay Dinshah, Roshan Dinshah, Alan Epstein, Ann Cottrell Free, Scott Frizlen, Brian Graff, Sharon Graff, Anne Green, Ph.D., Michael Greger, M.D., Alex Hershaft, Ph.D., Shirley Hunting, Brian Jacobs, Shari Kalina, Michael Klaper, M.D., Brian Klocke, Maureen Koplow, Howard Lyman, Karaena McCormack, Tahira McCormack, David Melina, Vesanto Melina, R.D., Ginny Messina, M.P.H., R.D., Eric Mills, Hillary Morris, Jack Norris, Larry Pearson, Marcia Pearson, Carl V. Phillips, M.P.P., Ph.D., Kevin Pickard, Tom Regan, Ph.D., Marianne Roberts, Julie Rosenfield, Rhoda Sapon, Stanley Sapon, Ph.D., Narendra Sheth, Sonal Sheth, David Shiller, Rae Sikora, David Smith, Kim Stallwood, Michael Stepaniak, Mae Lee Sun, Christina Vancheri, Shelton Walden, Zoe Weil, Judi Weiner, Bernie Wilke, Brad Wolff, and Kai Wu.

Several grassroots and national and international groups and organizations were instrumental in providing information, advocacy, guidance, and networking. They tirelessly toil every day to protect animals—the most exploited, abused, neglected, maligned, and murdered beings on Earth. This is emotionally taxing, heartbreaking, grueling, and typically thankless work. We owe them our deepest gratitude for persisting in this arduous task, in the face of constant defiance, pitted against a world filled with hostility, antagonism, and apathy. I urge you to support them in any way possible in their efforts to make this world a safer, saner, and more just place for all life:

Action for Animals

American Anti-Vivisection Society

American Fund for Alternatives to Animal Research

American Vegan Society

Animals' Agenda/Animal Rights Network

Beauty Without Cruelty USA

Center for Compassionate Living

Culture & Animals Foundation

Farm Sanctuary

Greyhound Friends, Inc.

Greyhound Protection League

HEART (Humans, the Environment and Animals Relating Together)

New England Anti-Vivisection Society

North American Vegetarian Society

PAWS (Performing Animal Welfare Society)

The Fund for Animals

Toronto Vegetarian Association

Vegan Foods, Inc., Designer Food Laboratories

United Poultry Concerns

The Vegan Society (England)

VEGAN ROOTS

People often say that humans have always eaten animals, as if this is a justification for continuing the practice. According to this logic, we should not try to prevent people from murdering other people, since this has also been done since earliest of times.

—Isaac Bashevis Singer

THE BIRTH OF A MOVEMENT

Long before the term *vegan* (pronounced VEE-gn) came into existence, there were individuals in the vegetarian movement who experimented with diets and lifestyles free from all products of animal origin. Often branded as extremists even by fellow vegetarians, these pioneers were few and far between and never formally organized as a group.

In July 1943, a letter from Leslie Cross appeared in *The Vegetarian Messenger,* the newsletter of the Leicester Vegetarian Society in England, expressing concerns about the use of dairy products by vegetarians. In March 1944, *The Vegetarian Messenger* published a summary of a lecture entitled "Should Vegetarians Eat Dairy Produce?" presented by Donald Watson at a society meeting in December 1943. In August 1944, Donald Watson and Elsie Shrigley discussed the desirability of forming a coalition of nondairy vegetarians. They approached the society to see if it would authorize such a subgroup and consign a page of *The Vegetarian Messenger* for them to express their views. Although sympathetic, the executive committee of the society rejected their proposal. In November 1944, Donald Watson, Elsie Shrigley, and five other interested people met at the Attic Club in Holborn, London, to discuss the name and formation of a new society. According to Elsie Shrigley, as reprinted in *The Vegan,* spring 1962, "It was a Sunday, with sunshine and a blue sky—an auspicious day for the birth of an idealistic movement."

WHAT'S IN A NAME?

Although some vegetarians have claimed that the word *vegetarian* is derived from the Latin *vegetus,* meaning "full of life," and not from the word *vegetable,* Donald Watson contends:

> The vegetarian movement has repeated this since its early days, and I suspect because of the frequent taunts that dairy produce and eggs can hardly be classed as vegetarian [coming from vegetables]. It has always seemed to me that this was a clever way to get round its critics.

The word *vegetarian* was defined in 1847 by the people who became the first members of the Vegetarian Society of Great Britain to describe individuals who would not eat meat, fowl, or fish. (Previously, those who abstained from eating meat were called Pythagoreans.) Donald Watson coined the word *vegan* when he grew tired of writing *total vegetarian* to describe vegetarians who do not use dairy products. The term prevailed over other suggestions at the time, including *dairybans, vitans, neovegetarians, benevores, bellevores, allvegas, sanivores,* and *beaumangeurs.* It was derived from the word *vegetarian* by taking the first three letters (*veg*) and the last two letters (*an*) because "veganism starts with vegetarianism and carries it through to its logical conclusion." As the originator of the word, Donald Watson, as quoted in *The Vegan,* spring 1989, is quite adamant that the pronunciation is with a long *e* and a hard *g*—not "veggan," "vaygun," "vayjun," or "veejun." The first published use of the word *vegan* was recorded in the *Oxford Illustrated Dictionary* in 1962.

Following are the dates when the term *vegan* has appeared in the *Oxford English Dictionaries* and how it has been defined:

- 1962—*Oxford Illustrated Dictionary*

  Vegetarian who eats no butter, eggs, cheese, or milk.
- 1973—*Shorter Oxford English Dictionary* (Addenda)

  A strict vegetarian; one who eats no animals or animal products.
- 1976—*Concise Oxford Dictionary* (7th ed.)

  [Person] eating no animals or animal products; strict[ly] vegetarian.
- 1986—*Oxford English Dictionary Supplement* (vol. 4)

  A person who on principle abstains from all food of animal origin; a strict vegetarian.
- 1989—*Oxford English Dictionary* (2d ed.)

  A person who on principle abstains from all food of animal origin; a strict vegetarian.
- 1993—*New Shorter Oxford English Dictionary*

  A total vegetarian, i.e., one who avoids dairy products and eggs as well as meat and fish.
- 1995—*Concise Oxford Dictionary* (9th ed.)

  A person who does not eat or use animal products.

THE PHOENIX RISES

After the Vegetarian Society rejected Donald Watson's proposal, he wrote a letter that outlined plans for a new society, which was printed in *The Vegetarian Messenger*. In response, thirty readers each sent him one shilling to cover the cost of the first four quarterly issues of a newsletter he offered to publish under the name *The Vegan News*.

This was a formidable time to initiate a new social movement. World War II was ending, shortages were rampant, and food rationing was at its most severe and would continue for another seven years. Vegetarians were successful in procuring extra cheese rations in place of meat, but vegans' attempts to obtain similar concessions were futile. There were no vegan cookbooks, and vitamin B_{12} had not yet been discovered. Some vegans did not fare well. Once the role of vitamin B_{12} was explored and better nutritional guidance was received, the situation for these determined trailblazers greatly improved.

Donald Watson commented in an article in *The Vegan,* summer 1988, entitled "Out of the Past," on why The Vegan Society was conceived during such a difficult period:

> Perhaps it seemed to us a fitting antidote to the sickening experience of the War, and a reminder that we should be doing more about the other holocaust that goes on all the time. Or perhaps it was that we were conscious of a remarkable omission in all previous vegetarian literature—namely, that though nature provides us with lots of examples of carnivores and vegetarians, it provides us with no examples of lacto-carnivores or lacto-vegetarians. Such groups are freaks and only made possible by man's capacity to exploit the reproductive functions of other species. This, we thought, could not be right either dietetically or ethically. It was certainly wrong aesthetically, and we could conceive of no spectacle more bizarre than that of a grown man attached at his meal-time to the udder of a cow.

EMANCIPATION PROCLAMATION

In November 1944, The Vegan Society published the following manifesto:

The Aims of The Vegan Society are:

(1) To advocate that man's food should be derived from fruits, nuts, vegetables, grains and other wholesome non-animal products and that it should exclude flesh, fish, fowl, eggs, honey, and animals' milk, butter, and cheese.

(2) To encourage the manufacture and use of alternatives to animal commodities.

The Vegan Society seeks to abolish man's dependence on animals, with its inevitable cruelty and slaughter, and to create instead a more reasonable and humane order of society. Whilst honouring the efforts of all who are striving to achieve the emancipation of man and of animals, The Vegan Society suggests that results must remain limited so long as the exploitation in food and clothing production is ignored.

The Vegan Society is eager that it should be realised how closely the meat and dairy produce industries are related. The atrocities of dairy farming are, in some ways, greater than those of the meat industry but they are more obscured by ignorance. Moreover, The Vegan Society asserts that the use of milk in any form after the period of weaning is biologically wrong and that, except when taken directly from the mother, it becomes polluted and unsafe. The Society, therefore, sees no honourable alternative but to challenge the traditions of orthodoxy by advocating a completely revised dietary based on reason and humane principle and guided by science and [designed] to meet physiological requirements.

It is not suggested that Veganism alone would be sufficient to solve all the problems of individual and social well-being, but so closely is its philosophy linked with morality, hygiene, aesthetics and agricultural economy that its adoption would remedy many unsatisfactory features of present-day life. Thus, if the curse of exploitation were removed, spiritual influences, operating for good, would develop conditions assuring a greater degree of happiness and prosperity for all.

This manifesto was especially significant because it called for the abolition not only of all foods of animal origin but of all animal-based commodities as well. Furthermore, it emphasized the moral, spiritual, social, health, and economic advantages of living by humane principles.

BEARING FRUIT

In the spring of 1946, the Leicester Vegetarian Society published *Vegetarian Recipes Without Dairy Produce,* by Margaret B. Rawls. That summer, The Vegan Society published its first cookbook, *Vegan Recipes,* by Fay K. Henderson. At the fall meeting, Donald Watson was elected the first president of The Vegan

Society, and the following day he accepted an offer to become the society's first life member.

In "The President's Log" of *The Vegan,* spring 1948, Donald Watson stated:

> The vegan case has proved itself impregnable against all reasonable criticism. The moral argument is so strong that no one dares to oppose it, and the physiological benefit is proved in practice. The economics of veganism are demonstrated to be sound by the fact that in time of economic crisis, nations tend to move toward vegan diets—the greater the crisis, the greater the move.

John Heron, then editor of *The Vegan,* wrote in the winter 1954–1955 issue:

> Veganism, startling and extreme to so many at its inception, now, after ten years, finds its ideals echoed throughout the world. Among a discerning minority in Europe, North America, in India and in Japan, the word "veganism" is known, its meaning and significance accepted and acknowledged.

WESTWARD, HO!

The emphasis of the British vegan movement was primarily on ethical concerns or, to use the phrase coined by Albert Schweitzer, "Reverence for Life" considerations. In the United States, interest in vegetarianism peaked during the mid-nineteenth century through the early part of the twentieth century, with the prevailing focus on health issues. Interest in vegetarian diets and diet reform in the United States declined toward the middle of the twentieth century. It was around this time that government organizations began producing and distributing food guides, all of which placed a heavy emphasis on meat and dairy products.

Nevertheless, a vegan movement had begun to take hold in the United States, albeit with little fanfare. As early as 1948, Dr. Catherine Nimmo, an ardent vegan since 1931 (more than a decade before the term was even created), and Rubin Abramowitz established this country's first Vegan Society, in Oceano, California, with encouragement and guidance from The Vegan Society in England. When Rubin Abramowitz moved back to Los Angeles, Nimmo, who had worked as the society's acting director, also took over the duties of acting secretary. She continued in this capacity until the incorporation of the American Vegan Society (AVS) by Jay Dinshah on February 8, 1960. Nimmo became AVS's first paying member.

FROM HUMBLE BEGINNINGS

Jay Dinshah had been a lifelong vegetarian. He had corresponded for quite a while with numerous vegetarian organizations around the world and had collected and studied a wide array of literature. When Jay received materials from The Vegan Society in England, however, he was surprised by what he discovered. Jay felt that if indeed the information he read was true, he had no choice but to become a vegan at once. He was not aware at the time of any health-related aspects of veganism; Jay's motivation was based strictly on ethics. In fact, Jay believed that regardless of the effects, "Life wasn't worth it if it depended on cruelty." Jay became a vegan in November 1957 at the tender age of twenty-four. At the age of twenty-six, Jay founded the American Vegan Society and established a historic presence for veganism in North America.

The American Vegan Society published its first issue of *Ahimsa* magazine in May 1960. It consisted of three single-sided pages printed on a hand-cranked mimeograph machine and bound with a staple. The annual membership fee was three dollars and included the monthly publication.

Ahimsa is a Sanskrit term that means nonharming, noninjuring. AVS defines it in modern terms as "dynamic harmlessness," implying that to follow the path of compassionate living requires practitioners not only to abstain from harming others but also to actively participate in providing protection, peace, and justice for all life. Each issue of *Ahimsa* delineates the six pillars of "the compassionate way." Combining the first letter of each pillar spells out the word *ahimsa*:

1. Abstinence from animal products.
2. Harmlessness with reverence for life.
3. Integrity of thought, word, and deed.
4. Mastery over oneself.
5. Service to humanity, nature, and creation.
6. Advancement of understanding and truth.

In August 1960, Jay Dinshah married 18-year-old Freya Smith from Epsom, England. A lifelong vegetarian and an ardent peace activist, she soon became corporate secretary of AVS. In September 1960, Freya, having become a vegan, composed her first *Ahimsa* article, entitled "A Step Further," where she stated:

> I have learned that the *moral* course is the one to be followed; the practical answers will be resolved once one opens his eyes sincerely. The full implication of moral, ethical vegetarianism cannot rest with just a renunciation of meat alone; it must go further and branch wider, finding full expression in the principles of Ahimsa and veganism.

From its inception, the American Vegan Society took a courageous stand against all forms of oppression, human *and* animal. An article by Jay Dinshah in the November 1960 issue of *Ahimsa* urged readers to employ their conscience in all matters of living:

> I do not believe that a conscience should be treated as the child of the mind, to be properly decorative, but not expected to express especially valuable opinions! Rather, it must be a constant guide for our everyday actions in our meetings with all creatures, human and otherwise.
>
> It is the primary function of this publication to arouse your thinking processes and encourage you to align your actions with the dictates of a fertile and active conscience. It is only when one stops repeating trite excuses and vain half-truths that one can really begin to hear the voice of conscience.
>
> Every day we are faced with many decisions of an ethical, moral nature—at every meal and in every business, personal,

and social transaction. Why do so many people thoughtlessly forfeit their own duty of conscience, surrendering to "convention" just because everyone else does it?

A February 1961 *Ahimsa* editorial, by Jay Dinshah, entitled "Let My People Go!" proclaimed:

> I call upon you, in the name of mercy and of justice, to speak out and to work for the eventual freedom of all creatures . . . to refuse to buy, sell, or utilize in any manner, shape or form any product of the cruelty, slavery, exploitation, pain, or death of an animal. . . .
>
> The cry for *freedom* and the right to live a peaceful life for oneself is formed on untold millions of mute tongues. If we who *can* speak for them remain silent, the very "stone will cry out of the wall!"

In that same issue, Catherine Nimmo expressed her view:

> Veganism is a practical expression of the Oneness of *all* Life. Veganism is basic, as it would not only do away with slaughter, vivisection, hunting, and fishing, but no doubt also with human exploitation.

In the March 1961 issue of *Ahimsa,* an article by Jay Dinshah entitled "What Would Happen If Everybody Practiced Complete Ahimsa?" declared:

> There is no peace through force or through fear. Unless Man learns to love his brother as himself, he will be left with neither brother nor self. The practice of Ahimsa is not a luxury, but an urgent worldwide necessity.

SPONTANEOUS GENERATION

By the early 1970s, there were a few existing religious sects that included some measure of vegetarian ideology and practice (Seventh-day Adventists, Theosophists, Buddhists, and others), and a few health-oriented organizations (the American Natural Hygiene Society, National Health Federation, etc.), but there was no secular nationwide vegetarian society. Around the turn of the century, the International Vegetarian Union (IVU) was established in Europe. Every two years or so, the IVU held meetings designated as World Vegetarian Congresses which convened in Europe or India. Since its inception in 1960, the American Vegan Society had sent representatives to every congress. When they inquired why a congress had never been held in the Western Hemisphere, the reply was that no organization had ever issued an invitation. In response, a formal invitation was presented at the 1973 congress in Sweden by AVS along with vegetarian representatives from Toronto, Montreal, and Los Angeles, and Helen and Scott Nearing of the Social Science Institute in Maine. The plan presented was essentially twofold: (1) to form a coast-to-coast umbrella organization to promote vegetarianism and encourage people to establish and operate local grassroots groups, and (2) to publicize, organize, and present the congress as a focal point for the renaissance of the vegetarian movement on the North American continent.

Freya and Jay Dinshah reflect that, in discussing this idea in a meeting with other IVU officials, Scott Nearing recalled (in what the Dinshahs describe as his "most tactful manner") that "We had a very good vegetarian convention in Lake Geneva, Wisconsin, in 1948. At the end of that we left it in the hands of [one of the organizers] to arrange another for the next year. That was twenty-five years ago, and we haven't heard any more about it since!" He expressed the view that the time was ripe for such a venture since there was so much new interest in vegetarianism. The IVU delegates voted overwhelmingly for this proposal, and an ad hoc committee held several planning meetings during the congress in Sweden.

The new umbrella organization was incorporated in early 1974 under the name of the North American Vegetarian Society (NAVS). Because the headquarters and staff of AVS were available to NAVS, the organization was able to immediately begin publishing a magazine called *Vegetarian Voice,* starting with the January/February 1974 issue. The initial aim was to encourage the growth of local vegetarian groups and get the word out about the World Vegetarian Congress planned for 1975, hosted by NAVS. The first issue was modest, but the second one included color photographs. With a press run of three hundred thousand, the magazine was distributed through health food stores, local groups, and a steadily growing mailing list, which eventually reached twenty thousand. By the time of the congress, more than one million copies of various eight-page, tabloid-size issues had been produced and distributed. They not only publicized the congress but also carried informative articles on all aspects of vegetarianism.

AVS recruited several idealistic and enthusiastic vegetarians to assist as volunteer workers to help make the congress a reality and take part in running it. Brian Graff, a valuable long-term volunteer, was named NAVS vice president. He also served for a decade as general secretary for the North American region of the International Vegetarian Union. Sharon Niblett arrived soon after Graff and was equally able and dedicated. They courted and married while living at the AVS headquarters, and their daughter Heidi was born there in 1976.

In addition to *Vegetarian Voice,* NAVS took on the responsibility of publishing the AVS booklet called *Facts of Vegetarianism,* which had an initial press run of forty thousand and a price of ten cents. NAVS brought out three more editions of the booklet, greatly enlarging it with nutrition information and two weeks' worth of vegan menus and recipes. By the time this publication was in its ninth edition, in 1982, the total number in print was two hundred thousand.

The January/February 1975 issue of *Vegetarian Voice* included a comprehensive guide entitled "How to Start a Local Vegetarian Society." Over the next year and a half, NAVS published four editions of the guide for a total of sixty-five thousand copies. The word was spreading and, by 1977, the roster of vegetarian groups in the United States and Canada had grown from six to about sixty. Over the years, the guide was revised and expanded. A fifth edition was printed in 1980, and the seventh edition appeared in AVS's *Ahimsa* magazine in 1999.

Over many months, NAVS assembled the recipes to be used for the 1975 World Vegetarian Congress. The recipes were all vegan and specifically tailored to suit a variety of tastes and dietary requirements. There was an intensive month of testing recipes initially designed to feed twenty to twenty-five people. Once the recipes were finalized, they were scaled up to feed one hundred and given to the University of Maine in Orono, where the congress was to be held. Here they were adjusted yet again to feed one thousand or more.

By congress time, NAVS had published a cookbook with the recipes in family-size portions. Later, after the book had been out of print for a decade, the recipes and menus were incorporated into the 1996 edition of Freya Dinshah's *The Vegan Kitchen* cookbook. The quantity-size recipes were published by NAVS in 1977 as a card file called "Vegetarian Cooking for 100," with a second printing the following year. Over the years, direct mail offers brought in thousands of orders from college campuses, prisons, restaurants, and local vegetarian groups. A newly revised edition was published by AVS in 1981.

After nearly two years of planning, preparing, and publicizing, the Twenty-third World Vegetarian Congress arrived at last on Western shores. It was held in August and ran for thirteen days. The first week was mainly educational featuring nearly ninety speakers from more than sixteen countries; the second week was more relaxed and informal. According to the Dinshahs, the congress "rode a rising tide of New Age interest and broke a long drought of veggie organization." The unprecedented publicity efforts were highly successful, attracting approximately fifteen hundred people to this momentous, groundbreaking event.

Attendees were invited to participate in an optional twenty-four-hour fast in symbolic sympathy with the hungry of the world. The university food service graciously agreed that the savings garnered from those who forfeited meals could be deducted from the total bill. The several hundred dollars raised from these efforts was forwarded to Vegfam, a British hunger-relief charity.

Afterward, a dramatic event was staged at the university's outdoor track, and again the focus was on feeding the world's hungry. The event included a mock "funeral for famine" using thousands of dollars' worth of borrowed equipment from a local funeral director. After the eulogy, volunteer pallbearers loaded the elegant and impressive (although empty) casket into a hearse.

News of the congress was covered by all three major television networks, and a CBS crew conducted on-campus interviews. Radio stations in cities as far away as San Diego learned about the congress via wire service and called the campus to do live or taped interviews. The largest and most prestigious U.S. newspapers and magazines, including the *New York Times, Washington Post, Washington Star, Philadelphia Inquirer,* and *Newsweek,* reported on the event, and even the international media (*International Herald Tribune* in

Milan, *Daily American* in Rome, *Ballymena Guardian* in Northern Ireland) reprinted the *New York Times* articles overseas.

Many people at the 1975 World Vegetarian Congress were notable vegetarian teachers. Some have since died: Henry Bailey Stevens, who wrote *The Recovery of Culture*; Richard St. Barbe Baker, author of *Sahara Conquest* and founder of Men of the Trees; Helen and Scott Nearing, distinguished pioneer homesteaders, ardent social reformers, prolific writers, and coauthors of the classic and beloved tome *Living the Good Life*; and Dr. Ann Wigmore, renowned advocate of wheat grass, sprouting, and raw foods. Others went on to become leaders in the worldwide vegan/vegetarian and animal rights movements: Pulitzer-nominated author and philosopher Tom Regan, Ph.D. (along with his wife, Nancy, and their children), who wrote the classic text *The Case for Animal Rights* and many other books and articles on animal rights; comedian, civil-rights activist, and author Dick Gregory; Alex Hershaft, Ph.D., founder of Farm Animal Reform Movement, author, and originator of numerous national vegetarian education campaigns and animal-rights conferences; Marcia Pearson, activist and organizer of Fashion with Compassion; journalist and poet Ann Cottrell Free, author of *No Room, Save in the Heart*; Frank and Rosalie Hurd, authors of the mostly vegan *Ten Talents* cookbook. Along with Australian philosopher Peter Singer's book *Animal Liberation,* which was published that same year, the 1975 World Vegetarian Congress was pivotal in inspiring and initiating the international crusade for animal rights.

The following year, NAVS organized a smaller, more streamlined, week-long convention at Ithaca College in New York. Subsequent annual conferences have been held in California, Rhode Island, Pennsylvania, Indiana, New Jersey, and again in New York. Eventually, the name was changed to the Vegetarian Summerfest. In 1984, NAVS again hosted the World Vegetarian Congress, this time in Catonsville, Maryland. It was the second time the congress had been held in the United States. Then, in 1996, NAVS joined once more with the International Vegetarian Union to present the Summerfest in conjunction with the World Vegetarian Congress in Johnstown, Pennsylvania. It was the first time the international congress had been on North American soil in more than a decade, and, at NAVS's insistence, it was *the first time* the meals at the event were totally vegan.

Unquestionably, the 1975 World Vegetarian Congress refocused and revitalized the vegetarian movement. Following are a few reminiscences from people who were there.

"Orono changed so many lives—I know it did mine." That was the first lady of vegetarianism in the nation's capital speaking: Madge Darneille. We were discussing the lasting impact of the World Vegetarian Congress held at the University of Maine at Orono nearly a quarter century earlier. The impact, we concluded, was not solely on one area of life, but many. That impact was broken into fragments as varied as the colorful chips of a kaleidoscope.

We remembered different things. I could see, for example, nearly fifteen hundred people standing in the cafeteria lines three times a day for meatless, dairyless meals, partaking of dishes little known to some of them. For many, it was a first encounter with veganism that sent some back to the line for seconds!

Little things stand out. Enormous platters of fresh ears of corn. Uncooked and delicious! The various uses of the magical soybean and the healthful power of garlic. (A vigorous, eightyish lady from Finland gave daily garlic cloves credit for her overwhelming energy.)

We could hear men and women from California, New York, England, India, Canada, Finland, Ireland, and numerous other states and countries—whether in the dining room, on campus, or in classroom sessions—exchanging new ideas about food, health, children, and animals.

We could see many of us crowded into the kitchen of the revered Scott and Helen Nearing, who lived nearby and who were partially responsible for the conference being held at Orono. We remember the taste and the aroma of the enormous pot of soup concocted by Helen from their own vegetables and herbs. And her home-baked multigrain bread—well, words fail.

We marveled at the miracle they had wrought in their garden, which had been brought to fruitfulness by their hard work and enrichment of hard, rocky soil. At that time, radical writer, philosopher, labor leader Scott Nearing was in his nineties and musician-writer Helen Nearing was in her seventies.

A year earlier Helen and Scott Nearing had met with Madge, Brian Graff, Ben Weiss, Sig Linnio, Jay and Freya Dinshah, International Vegetarian Union president Gordon Latto and general secretary Brian Gunn-King, professor Henry Bailey Stevens, and several others, to plan the surprisingly successful conference. Madge was the president of the Vegetarian Society of Washington, D.C., and the Dinshahs were leaders of the American Vegan Society. It was at that time that the North American Vegetarian Society was born and the Orono conference was on its way!

No one attending the conference could ever forget the Dinshahs' dedication and resourcefulness in masterminding the conference—from Freya in the kitchen to Jay all over the lot! The timing was right. In the early 1970s, conscious revolt against meat-and-gravy life was getting underway, as well as concern about the exploitation of animals raised for food.

Lives were changed for a variety of philosophical and health reasons. But perhaps the main reason for the success of Orono was the realization that we were not alone and that we were in the vanguard of a healthier future no longer based on enslavement of other beings.

—ANN COTTRELL FREE

I remember the wonderful feeling of being surrounded by so many vegetarians. I had only been veggie for about a year and a half, so I was not aware that there were so many ways to be vegetarian. I had made the choice because of my love for animals and the realization that eating meat actually meant eating animal bodies. The switch that clicked for me was sudden and irrevocable. But it simply meant that I no longer ate animals. It was a "negative" reaction in that it only encompassed what I would not do. The finer points, such as all the new foods that I would eat, were not obvious to me at the time.

At the congress I discovered entirely new ingredients and expanded cuisines. Although there were many speakers and workshops on the health aspects of vegetarianism, I did not pay much attention to them.

Personal health benefits that come from avoiding flesh are a bonus and are certainly welcome. But I would avoid flesh even if the only benefit was a clear conscience. I felt that way when I first stopped eating animals, and that was my philosophy when I attended the congress. Fortunately, there were also speakers and workshops that dealt with my concerns. And, in spite of my own single-mindedness, I was awestruck by the multiplicity of reasons for eschewing (not chewing) meat.

—MAUREEN KOPLOW

By the spring of 1975, I had been a closet vegetarian for thirteen years and had never known any other vegetarians. When I came across a leaflet promoting the World Vegetarian Congress scheduled that summer in Orono, Maine, I felt that this would be a good opportunity to determine whether the time had arrived to come out of the closet. Indeed, seeing fifteen hundred vegetarians from different parts of the world, with different professions and education levels, wearing different clothes and speaking different tongues, was my epiphany. I decided right then and there to come out of the closet and to just keep on going, devoting the rest of my life to the promotion of meatless eating.

—ALEX HERSHAFT

While nurturing the growth of NAVS and organizing the congresses, AVS had sacrificed so much time and effort that its own needs were suffering. Its membership had dwindled and *Ahimsa* had shrunk to only one magazine issue per year. It was time for an amicable separation.

Brian and Sharon Graff moved to Dolgeville, New York, and set up the NAVS headquarters there, where it has become a thriving organization. In addition to coordinating the annual Summerfest conferences—which feature premier speakers and leaders in the vegan/vegetarian, animal-rights, and environmental movements and attract attendees from around the world—NAVS continues to distribute literature and vegetarian support materials to individuals and grassroots vegetarian groups across North America. It also produces the quarterly *Vegetarian Voice* magazine along with numerous other pamphlets and publications. Although founded and rooted as a vegetarian umbrella group, most of NAVS's leaders happened to be vegan; consequently, the organization has maintained a decidedly vegan bent. In the early 1980s, the NAVS board of trustees established the official policy that no recipes using animal foods or ingredients would be served at any NAVS events or published in *Vegetarian Voice,* or in any other NAVS publications.

After the NAVS move, the American Vegan Society redirected its energies. Without missing a beat, it continues to serve as a fountain of knowledge, understanding, and inspiration for individuals and groups around the world. AVS also sponsors an annual convention where vegan leaders, professionals, and educators share their wisdom and experience with supporters from all across the North American continent. *Ahimsa* has expanded into a twenty-four-page quarterly magazine, and the Society continues to produce numerous pamphlets and publications including Freya's landmark book *The Vegan Kitchen,* first published in 1965 and now in its thirteenth printing.

Since the founding of AVS and NAVS, countless vegan and animal rights groups have proliferated throughout the world. In 1980, the formation of People for the Ethical Treatment of Animals (PETA) helped establish a very public case for a diet and lifestyle based on humane concerns. Once considered an insignificant "fringe group of fanatics," vegans today are viewed as the vanguard of the vegetarian, animal rights, and humane movements. In correspondence to Freya Dinshah dated July 4, 1997, Donald Watson stated:

> It is a profound thought that we may have cracked the code that has beaten everyone else to show how mankind can live in a state of health and harmony and that all others have merely been tinkering with the problem.

2

THE VEGAN IDENTITY

There is so much in this world that most people just never see anymore. It is sad knowing that they can go through life never realizing what treasures we have before us. I think this is the main reason people have become so numb to their feelings—why compassion is a stranger. If people could only see, they would understand.

—KEVIN PICKARD

IN SEARCH OF SELF

Vegans are a heterogeneous group and cannot be categorized by age, race, gender, ethnicity, ability, religion, income, sexual orientation, educational level, or physical traits. Vegans work in a wide variety of fields and occupations and can be found in all parts of the world.

Because vegans cannot be identified by appearance, they are often isolated from each other both professionally and socially. Although they are united by a shared ethic, the only distinguishing characteristic vegans have is their behavior—the active application of their ethic. This is called *veganism* (pronounced VEE-gn-izm). The American Vegan Society defines veganism as follows:

> Veganism means living solely on the products of the plant kingdom, to the exclusion of flesh, fish, fowl, animal milk, and all dairy products (cheese, butter, yogurt, etc.), eggs, honey, and all other foods of animal origin.

19

It also excludes from use animal products such as fur, wool, leather, and silk, notably items of clothing. Vegans also usually make efforts to avoid various less-than-obvious animal secretions, oils, etc., used in many cosmetics, toiletries, household goods, and other everyday commodities. Veganism encourages finding and using alternatives for these and all other materials from animal sources. Vegans may be described as those who have taken the next logical ethical steps beyond basic vegetarianism.

Based on this definition, the practice of veganism entails abstaining from the use of all animal products in every aspect of daily living, from personal-care items and cleaning products to clothing, jewelry, and footwear. Veganism is not merely passive resistance. It compels practitioners to find alternatives to commodities typically made from animal products or by-products and to make deliberate and dynamic choices about each and every activity in their lives.

INVESTIGATING THE OBSCURE

The definition presented by AVS focuses specifically on the *behavior* that delineates a vegan. It does not consider motive, nor does it address moral, religious, or spiritual convictions. It does not judge practitioners' activities. It does not explore or prescribe belief systems for practitioners. The implication of this definition is succinct: A vegan is characterized not by what he or she *believes* but by what he or she *does*. In other words, it is not enough to have right *thought*; to be vegan one must have right *action*.

Nevertheless, most nonvegans are curious what would prompt someone to adopt a position so contrary to mainstream views, a lifestyle that, to many, would seem destined to invoke challenge and adversity. Catherine Nimmo, quoted in the April/June 1985 issue of *Ahimsa,* said:

> If we become vegans because we understand animals and feel great compassion for their sufferings, it is the easiest thing, and proves to be of the greatest benefit for ourselves too; but if we become vegans for health reasons, it seems full of worries based on fear, ignorance, and above all egocentric thinking.

WHERE THERE IS SMOKE

The revelation that it is unethical, immoral, inhumane, sinful, or karmically wrong to participate in any way in the killing, suffering, or unjust control of animals can change lives forever. Those who are brought to veganism through ethical or spiritual guidelines are most likely to maintain their beliefs even in an unsupportive society. Generally, this is because these vegans determine that intuitive moral codes take precedence over cultural dicta. Vegans who practice an ethical standard based on deeply held principles in lieu of following preordained societal norms find maintaining their veganism relatively effortless and the thought of returning to the use of animal products impossible and ignoble.

Although health considerations may be a motivating factor for some individuals to become total vegetarians (those who avoid all animal products in diet only), it is generally insufficient incentive for the elimination of animal products from other parts of one's life. Because veganism encompasses all aspects of daily living, not just diet, it is completely inaccurate for people to define themselves as such simply because they have adopted the vegan mode of eating. Practicing a vegan diet no more qualifies someone as vegan than eating kosher food qualifies someone as Jewish.

Most people who come to vegetarianism (let alone veganism) for the sole purpose of improving their health have little reason to make a long-term commitment, unless, of course, the diet makes them feel better or reverses or improves an ailment. If, however, a new animal-based product was touted as the best remedy for their particular affliction, and it could not be made from plant material or manufactured synthetically, there is little doubt the attraction would be irresistible. Furthermore, there is simply no inducement for the strictly health-motivated vegetarian to seek out vegan clothing, cosmetics, or household products.

Occasionally what occurs is a transformation, an evolution of one's initial stimulus over a period of time. Some people may become vegetarians for health objectives and discover a host of other reasons that further justify their choice. These may ultimately direct them toward veganism, and additional realizations may strengthen their resolution.

David Melina, a seventeen-year vegan, witnessed the early death of his father from cancer and saw his mother endure breast cancer and an untimely death from adult-onset diabetes, diseases he believes were diet related. He was propelled to vegetarianism and later to veganism because of these experiences and growing concerns about his own physical health. Today, however, David's motivation is quite different. This shift in viewpoint is not uncommon among those drawn to veganism for issues pertaining to health.

> I have learned a great deal over the years about the cruelty that is inflicted on animals in food and clothing production, entertainment, education, and experimentation, and how our dependence on animal and chemical agriculture is polluting our environment, depleting resources, destroying rain forest and wildlife habitat, and exploiting many people in Third World countries. For me, it's not just the health issue anymore.

Kevin Pickard experienced a similar evolution:

> Over time I became aware—ironically, for the *first* time—of the ethical reasons for a vegan diet. Like most people in our society, I had never made the connection between the animals and the "food" we eat. I think these reasons took the longest for me to adopt. From my experience, I think most people become vegan for ethical reasons first and then the other reasons follow. I started out from the other end, with a concern for myself. It wasn't until later that I expanded my circle of compassion to include others. I began to see the insanity and cruelty in the way we treat those with whom we share the planet.

TRUTH OR CONTROVERSY

We all occasionally make decisions that confound logic—our choice of a mate, our musical preferences, our taste in clothing, our hobbies and interests. As much as we might try to defend our predilections, there is no deductive way to explain them. They are simply a part of us, the special attributes that make each of us uniquely ourselves. Few of us relish the idea that our propensities may be the result of cultural conditioning—that we are products of our environment and not the other way around.

Numerous influences contribute to the development of our tastes, outlook, and beliefs, which combine to create our worldview—"truths" we accept, take for granted, and rarely challenge. For instance, you may "know" that looking someone in the eye is a sign of honesty, but in some cultures, it is a sign of disrespect. Who is right? It all depends on your worldview—your cultural upbringing and your beliefs.

Questioning our worldview is a difficult, sometimes impossible task. There are so many elements in our lives that we just assume to be correct that it usually doesn't even occur to us to question them. Even when pressured by outside forces, we tend to cling to our own worldview rather than consider other perspectives. That is why choosing to be vegan can seem so enigmatic to friends, family, and coworkers. Challenging the validity of accepted societal norms makes people uneasy. It brings up issues most people never think about, let alone want to talk about.

If, for example, a young woman confronts her parents about the impropriety of eating meat or wearing leather shoes, it might very well be interpreted as a direct challenge to their personal values. After all, they have always eaten meat and worn leather shoes, as have their parents and their parents before them. If they were to renounce eating meat and wearing leather shoes, in what ways would their lives be changed, and would these changes be acceptable or intolerable? How would it affect them socially and professionally? What would it imply for the mores and customs they have practiced all their lives? Could their daughter's words imply that she thinks of them as ignorant, immoral, or irrational people who blindly follow a baseless set of precepts without question? Brian Klocke came face-to-face with this situation:

> I grew up in Iowa as a Catholic on a family farm that raised pigs and cattle for slaughter and corn and soybeans for animal feed. When I was very young, we butchered chickens. I also participated in hunting and trapping as a farm kid. It has been difficult coming to terms with some of the violence I committed and some of the violence I saw family members committing toward animals. I am the only vegetarian and vegan in my immediate family, and I know of only one other vegetarian (not vegan) in the group of more than a hundred first cousins I am related to.

Not only were my parents animal and grain farmers (they are retired now), but their parents were as well, in addition to all their friends. My becoming vegan was very difficult for my family to handle at first and thus made my interactions with them difficult as well. At first, I did everything I could to not bring up the subject of veganism. When I was asked why I was vegan and I explained a few of my reasons, including compassion for animals, my family immediately became defensive. It was as if I had rejected their very livelihood and the values that they had instilled in me.

Most of us prefer to navigate through life with as few bumps and curves as possible. Change and challenge can be unpleasant, so we generally opt to avoid them whenever we can. Choosing to become vegan can throw a major kink into someone's life. What could persuade someone to make such a drastic metamorphosis?

> It is said that once you look behind the curtain, you cannot pretend you do not know what is behind the curtain. Behind the curtain marked VEGAN in my mind are the eyes of all the animals of the world, all the children of the world, and all the unborn souls to come—each watching my every choice and every action. My love for them leaves me no choice but to be vegan—from moment to moment, decision after decision, as the years go by. As our society's exploitative use of animals becomes more evident, I must acknowledge them and align my actions accordingly.
>
> I have parted the curtain wide, and now there is no pretending that I do not know—there is no going back. I have been an orthodox vegan for the past sixteen years and cannot conceive of continuing my life span on this earth in any other manner.
>
> —MICHAEL KLAPER

TINTING THE LENS

Western cultures are made up of two worlds—that which is seen and that which is hidden from view. When something is concealed, there is rarely cause to think about it. "Out of sight, out of mind" is a widely accepted credo.

History is replete with examples of worldviews that today would be considered taboo, unthinkable. For example, not all that long ago, men and women of African descent and other people of color in the United States were regarded as slaves and property. Few whites viewed brown- and black-skinned people otherwise. The worldview the whites subscribed to espoused that people of color, simply by virtue of having darker skin, were inferior and somehow less human. This worldview enabled them to commit unspeakable atrocities that today would be considered immoral. Yet the whites who enslaved Africans rationalized their actions with platitudes like "They were raised for that." This type of commentary perpetuated the illusion that living beings, human or otherwise, who are raised for a particular purpose should not mind their destiny, that the abuse and suffering inflicted on them should somehow be more easily tolerated and exonerated. If individuals are viewed as dissimilar from and therefore unequal to those in power, abuse and torture can be conveniently sanctioned, perhaps even encouraged, especially if it benefits the power holders.

Despite significant changes in federal law and public policy, racism remains rampant. It is a horrifying and blatant example of how tenacious worldviews can be, and how the attitudes and myths they proliferate are so utterly resistant to change.

A similar worldview can be seen in Nazi Germany's obliteration of millions of Jewish men, women, and children; homosexuals; gypsies; social outcasts; and dissenters. The Nazi officers were able to discharge their heinous crimes by accepting a worldview that designated certain individuals as subhuman and therefore deserving of extermination. When brought to trial for committing crimes against humanity, these men asserted they were only doing their jobs.

These examples of mass enslavement, torture, and slaughter epitomize the depths to which humanity will sink if it adopts a worldview accepting of these horrors. Those wielding the power didn't regard their acts as abominable or nefarious; they perceived them as justifiable, necessary, even beneficial. Whites who massacred Native Americans or enslaved and murdered Africans, as well as Nazis who exterminated Jews, held a worldview that didn't see the intrinsic value of those they persecuted; hence they committed their atrocities without remorse.

When dominant human groups define themselves as superior to groups they wish to subordinate, they draw specific distinctions. For instance, whites define people of color by the differing melanin content of their skin, and men distinguish women by primary and secondary sex characteristics. These empirical differences are then used to "justify" social dominance of one group over the other even though it is the *social interpretation* of these distinctions, not the distinctions themselves, that serve to keep one group on top.

The distinctions between human and nonhuman animals are used in the same fashion. Characteristics that distinguish other animals from humans are ranked and classified; those characteristics that are most unlike our own are then used to explain the supposed inferiority of other animals. There is tremendous absurdity in exclusionary/inclusionary systems that are built around inconsequential attributes and designed solely for the purpose of supporting self-serving theories.

When there is a supposed benefit to be gained by treating animals as we do—exploiting their labor, eating their bodies, gawking at them, or owning them as a sign of social status—we see them as slaves, food, entertainment, or property, not as living, sensate individuals. This view is integrated into our cultural mores, even promoted. We try to justify our "right" to dominate other animals by their differences—their so-called lesser characteristics. Speciesism can certainly be compared with other forms of bigotry. Fundamental prejudice is at the core of racism, sexism, *and* speciesism.

> Racists are people who think that the members of their race are superior to the members of other races simply because the former belong to their (the "superior") race. Sexists believe that the members of their sex are superior to the members of the opposite sex simply because the former belong to their (the "superior") sex. Both racism and sexism are paradigms of insupportable bigotry. There is no superior or inferior sex or race. Racial and sexual differences are biological, not moral. The same is true of speciesism—the view that members of the species Homo sapiens *are superior to members of every other species simply because human beings belong to one's own (the "superior") species. For there is no superior species. To think otherwise is to be no less prejudiced than racists or sexists.*
>
> —TOM REGAN

LIVING ON THE EDGE

My most difficult challenge is the world of human indifference. It is standing in line at the supermarket and realizing that for the majority of people in the world, the misery and slaughter of animals is not an issue.

—KAREN DAVIS

There is a saying that goes as follows: "If slaughterhouses had glass walls, everyone would become a vegetarian." This epigram is reflective of several worldviews maintained by Western industrialized cultures and carefully cultivated by the meat, dairy, and egg industries. First, we can find in it the implication that slaughterhouses (euphemistically called processing plants or packing plants) are camouflaged, that perhaps people aren't even aware of their existence. Second, they are places where activities are well concealed. And third, these activities necessitate obscurity because they are so totally revolting that, if seen, they would immediately transform onlookers.

Most people never think about how their meat gets to the supermarket. They don't see the slaughterhouse physically because it isn't located in the center of town, and its facade is typically disguised. They don't see it in their mind's eye either. To visualize the screams, death, and dismemberment of the animals whose flesh is in the cellophane-wrapped packages in their supermarket's cooler would be too painful and upsetting for most people to bear. It is easier, perhaps, to accept a worldview that, although rife with lies, tells us the animals were raised by kind, caring farmers in the bucolic countryside where they grazed and propagated freely and died of natural causes.

Few meat eaters concede the reality that the majority of the nearly nine billion animals raised and slaughtered for food each year in the United States alone are cruelly confined in appalling factory farms; subjected to dreadful surgeries and tortures including mutilations and amputations without anesthesia; artificially inseminated; genetically manipulated; brutally transported; and barbarously killed. Those who are consciously aware of the facts most often appease their conscience by telling themselves that these abominations can't be helped because meat is a necessary evil, or that it's essential to maintain good health, or that the government wouldn't let this happen, or that the animals are raised for this, so it's okay, or hundreds of other prevarications that are corroborated by meat-industry ads and promotions, governmental agencies, and misguided health-care workers.

What would transpire if the public allowed itself to hear the cries of the animals, witness the bloodshed, and admit that there is a war being waged right on our own soil, right in our own backyard, right this very minute? It would be a frightening acknowledgment, because previous silences could be interpreted as admissions of guilt, implying a level of complicity or at least culpability. Furthermore, this heightened awareness would oblige moral meat eaters to make serious modifications in their diets and their lives. Sadly, many people would prefer to live in denial than take the time and trouble to change.

> *While I had long enjoyed the taste of meat, especially beef and even veal, it always disturbed me to go to the butcher shop, especially those in Chinatown where euphemisms for animal products are fewer than in Western supermarkets. So constant denial of the truth was essential for my earlier dietary habits. After I learned of the torture of animals, the sellout of our health, and the poisoning of our earth, denial became untenable—indeed, it would have been monstrous.*
>
> —KAI WU

Matt Ball, a doctoral candidate in environmental engineering, remembers his first encounter with vegetarianism, during his freshman year in college. He recollects his roommate playing music by the Smiths and the simple, undeniable logic of the lyrics on *Meat Is Murder*: "It's death for no reason, and death for no reason is murder." His roommate was a vegetarian.

> What could I do? My head knew that this was true, and my heart was repulsed at the thought of factory farms and slaughterhouses. Meat is murder, and it is wrong. Yet my traditions—everything I had been taught to believe and to honor—said that eating meat, animals, was okay, unquestionably accepted and inherently good. To listen to my own thoughts and decide for myself would be to reject the central celebration of meat by my friends and family, for I knew that once I accepted the cruelty

and cut meat from my diet, it would not be okay to be around others and remain silent, as if nothing were amiss, as if nothing had changed. To this day, I dread discussing vegetarianism. Since I met my roommate ten years ago, I have seen factory farms and been to slaughterhouses; the screams of these animals stay with me every day. It is the worst when I am faced with someone who reacts as I once reacted—not wanting to hear, not wanting to question, not wanting to change. The agonies of the animals, living and dying hidden from our eyes and ears, their corpses disguised and exalted on our plates, struggle against my sympathy for the person confronted and my desire to avoid judgment. While I try to be moderate and reasonable, I know that eating meat is not a matter of choice any more than slavery or child abuse is a matter of choice. It is the exploitation and murder of fellow sentient beings who feel pain and fight to stay alive. In the face of this injustice and suffering, of what compulsion is conformity?

EXTENDING THE CIRCLE

If we pay attention, humans can easily identify the signs of suffering in other species. We exhibit many of the same behaviors, so it is logical to assume that many of our feelings are similar. We cannot prove that other humans feel pain or any other emotion the same as we do, yet we do not doubt that their emotional experiences are as real and valid as our own. There is no logical rationale—scientific, moral, or philosophical—for denying the sensate lives of animals. If we concede that other humans feel pain, we must concede that other animals do as well. Indeed, scientific responsibility obligates us to accept, on faith, the existence of other animals' emotional lives, even if we do not fully comprehend their depth or modes of expression.

Although the majority of scientists prefer not to acknowledge the feelings of animals for fear of anthropomorphizing them, anyone who has ever lived among cats or dogs can attest to their wide range of emotions and describe how they exhibit joy, excitement, sadness, and fear. If the explanation for these emotions is that they are merely anthropomorphic projection, it is an incredibly pervasive delusion.

People who have spent time among farm animals recognize these same emotional attributes in pigs, cows, sheep, goats, turkeys, and chickens. Although each species has its own unique way of communicating its needs and feelings, it takes only a brief time for the careful observer to discern what is being conveyed. And just like dogs and cats, just like all living creatures including ourselves, each farm animal has a unique personality, with preferences, habits, and quirks that distinguish one individual from the next.

Vegans subscribe to an alternative worldview that recognizes that all animals exist for their own purposes, feel pain, and suffer. Therefore, it is unconscionable to usurp or manipulate their lives or impose suffering upon them for our own pleasure or gain regardless of any perceived value or advantage to humans.

When we consider the horrors that people perpetrate on each other despite our cognizance of human suffering, we can draw many parallels between our victimization of other humans and our exploitation of animals. Brian Graff awoke to this realization while serving in the military during the early 1970s.

> Having grown up with a softhearted feeling toward animals, I found it was an easy decision to become vegan. The idea that you could live without eating animals or exploiting them for commodities struck a chord within me. It made clear and immediate sense. At the dawn of my awakening, it so amazed me that I had not heard about vegetarianism or veganism before in my twenty-one years. The transition to veganism came on the heels of my having decided that I wanted no part in killing humans directly or indirectly. This was not a popular position to take, considering I was at the time serving in the U.S. Navy and involved in a secret intelligence operation. By the time I applied for a conscientious-objector discharge from the military, I had come to see the killing of humans and other animals as one and the same.

The analogy between human and animal suffering also had a particularly profound meaning for Alex Hershaft, who immigrated to the United States from Poland and Italy in 1951.

My experiences in the Warsaw Ghetto during the Holocaust had a profound impact on my subsequent life choices. I felt some guilt that I lived when so many others didn't and a sense of duty to redeem my survival by assuming their share of responsibility for making this planet a better place to live for all its inhabitants.

After the war, I became active in the religious freedom, civil rights, peace, and environmental movements, receiving much fulfillment but always feeling that I was missing something. Following my deeply emotional experience at the World Vegetarian Congress in 1975, I took time to reflect on the root of the key problems challenging planetary survival, i.e. disease, hunger, environmental devastation, oppression, and war. Amazingly, all evidence pointed to animal agriculture as the common root cause. My life's mission then became crystal clear.

In particular, my experiences in the Nazi Holocaust allowed me to empathize with the condition of farm animals in today's factory farms, auction yards, and slaughterhouses. I know first-hand what it's like to be treated like a worthless object, to be hunted by the killers of my family and friends, to wonder each day if I will see the next sunrise, to be crammed in a cattle car on the way to slaughter.

THE WAY THE WEST WAS WEANED

Why would it be necessary for human beings to drink the milk of another mammal to be healthy? A mother cow's milk is designed specifically for her calf; likewise, a human mother's milk is designed specifically for a human baby. Does the calf have to drink the human mother's milk to be healthy? If not, then why should a human being drink the milk of a cow to be healthy?

—JEFFREY BROWN

EMBRACING THE ABSURD

Western culture has been conditioned through incredibly effective promotional campaigns, promulgated by the self-serving interests of the dairy industry, to believe that bodily fluids discharged from cows' udders are not only tasty, nutritious, and wholesome but also an absolute necessity for sound human health. Through carefully conceived marketing tactics and powerful lobbying efforts, the majority of consumers, educators, and health-care practitioners have been seduced into viewing cow's milk as the singular source of dietary calcium, the perfect food for children, and the only way women can thwart osteoporosis. It has seemed irrelevant to most North Americans that many plant foods have as much calcium as cow's milk and some have even more, with drastically lower fat, no cholesterol, significantly greater overall nutrition, and an abundance of antioxidants and fiber, which have both been shown to help stave off some cancers and other illnesses. Furthermore, despite the utter preposterousness of a person being suckled by a cow, the dairy industry has duped the public into believing that cow's milk is a completely natural food for human beings.

There is a simple absurdity in the human consumption of cow's milk. All other mammals consume their mother's milk as infants and are eventually weaned, usually after they have tripled their birth weight. Their mother's milk is nutritionally balanced in fat, protein, and other nutrients for the proper development of that particular species' young. Humans, however, are an anomaly, being the only species of mammal that is never weaned. No other mammals continue to drink milk after the weaning stage and certainly never through adulthood. But even more peculiar is that no mammals in their natural environment other than human beings take the milk of another species.

Of course, it is not in the financial interest of the dairy industry to point out these facts. The mission of their trade organizations is to present milk and dairy products in the best light possible so that society will remain dependent on milk, cheese, ice cream, and sundry other dairy foods as dietary staples, and revenues will continue to swell. Cow's milk and dairy products have not only infiltrated our kitchens, they have so permeated our cultural practices that they have in essence become a socially acceptable and encouraged psychological addiction. In light of the beef-eating public's apathetic response to the threat of mad cow disease in England and the deadly *E. coli* bacteria in the United States, it is exceedingly unlikely that habits will change, even if consumers were confronted with serious health risks from cow's milk. This is how commanding the dairy industry's grip is over the public appetite.

Milk consumption is a distinct example of a worldview out of control. Dairy products have become such an integral part of our cuisine and customs that anyone who dares spurn them is viewed with skepticism or deemed un-American. Thus, challenging the merits and ethicalness of consuming such a beloved and seemingly indispensable product is a daunting task for vegans.

BEHIND THE BARN DOOR

It is obvious even to the casual bystander that before the flesh of an animal can be procured for human consumption the animal must first be killed. Because of this, even some meat eaters can be sympathetic to the vegetarian cause in spite of their own reluctance to stop eating meat. What is not so evident, however, is why vegans also avoid eating other animal products, such as cow's milk and eggs, which can ostensibly be produced without causing death.

As with stockyards, slaughterhouses, and meat packing plants, dairy processors rarely show what they don't want consumers to see or know. Advertisements emphasize the salable attributes of products; information that is less than respectable is hidden from the public eye. Understandably, dairy farmers want the public to desire their products and feel good about using them. As a result, the dairy industry has painted a utopian but highly fallacious image of modern dairy production. Impressions aside, dairying is big business. And as with all business, interests boil down to the bottom line.

MILK, MONEY, AND MADNESS

More milk means more money. Therefore, milk production is augmented by a variety of spurious means, including intensive factory-style farming where the standard modus operandi includes the use of hormones and drugs. Artificial insemination is endemic; *Scientific Farm Animal Production,* an industry textbook, explains that approximately 70 percent of dairy cows and 25 percent of heifers are bred artificially. Genetic manipulation is customary and rampant. Industrywide, it is affirmed that the primary goal of a breeding program should be to produce cows with the greatest possible genetic capacity to make a profit.

The unmitigated desire for greater revenue has driven the dairy industry to employ numerous invidious techniques, with little concern for the comfort or well-being of the cows. The objective is simply to drain as much profit from each animal, regardless of how callous the methods may be. As a result, today's modern dairy cow is a freakish amalgam of unnatural parts. In *Understanding the Dairy Cow,* an industry text, John Webster observes that the selection of dairy cows for increased yield has produced big, angular animals with large, over-distended udders and distorted hind legs, further exacerbating the problems of standing, walking, and especially lying on hard surfaces.

This mad-scientist approach to dairy production has created a monster cow who, according to the USDA national agricultural statistics on milk production, currently yields about 45 pounds of milk per day, significantly more than she would produce in nature. By comparison, USDA statistics reveal that milk production for the average dairy cow in 1960 was only about 20 pounds per day. As a result of this outrageous increase, cows' bodies are under constant stress and at risk for numerous infections, diseases, and other health problems. The USDA's "Dairy Management Practices" report indicates that approximately one in seven dairy cows in the United States suffers from clinical mastitis, a painful bacterial infection of the udders that is exacerbated by accelerated milk production. In advanced stages, mastitis can be fatal; it is the second leading cause of death in dairy cows who die prior to slaughter. Mastitis, termed a "production disease," is one of the most frequent and costly afflictions in intensive dairy production. In fact, mastitis is, and has been, such a common and financially catastrophic ailment that the dairy industry established the National Mastitis Council in 1961 specifically to study and combat this disease.

In a natural environment, a cow would spend her days foraging, ruminating, and caring for her young, typically allowing her calf to suckle as often as he or she desired. On modern dairy farms, however, cows are viewed first and foremost as milking machines. Their normal needs and inclinations are disregarded or forcibly squelched. Dairy cows are commonly housed in cramped, narrow concrete stalls or storage cages for nearly ten months out of the year. In general, the only time the cows are allowed to emerge is when they are milked by electric contraptions two or three times a day. John Webster, in *Understanding the Dairy Cow,* points out the implicit absurdity of breeding a cow capable of producing huge quantities of milk per day and then restricting her to only two milkings instead of the five to seven feedings she would normally indulge her calf. He adds that this is yet another contributor to udder distension, which subsequently leads to more mastitis and lameness.

SUCKED DRY

Although most North Americans envision dairy cows living in comfort and grazing on grassy knolls in the countryside, the truth is that about a quarter of all dairy cows have no access to the outdoors. A survey conducted over several years by a Holstein trade organization revealed that the majority of herds in winter spend nearly the entire day and night on concrete, with about 25 percent of these cows having less than an hour of exercise per day. Additionally, the survey found that over half of all herds year-round are kept in tie stalls, as opposed to free stalls or loose housing. Nevertheless, the myth of the contented dairy cow, as promoted by industry representatives, persists.

On a normal grass diet, cows would be unable to produce milk at the extraordinarily high levels demanded by modern dairies. Therefore, dairy cows are given rich, high-energy feeds. But these can cause serious metabolic disorders, including ketosis, which can be fatal, and laminitis, a painful inflammation of the hoof. Foot lameness, an increasing problem, has been attributed to changes in physical conformation imposed by selective breeding, abnormally rich nutrition, lack of exercise, and extended periods in uncomfortable housing, all engineered in the interest of improved productivity and profit. Another common dairy-industry disease is milk fever, an ailment caused by calcium deficiency, which occurs when milk production depletes calcium faster than it can be replenished in the cow's blood.

Of course, the dairy industry is well aware of these and other health problems associated with intensive milk production. It also recognizes the need for farmers to protect their financial investments. However, when mistreating animals is profitable, it becomes the industry norm. As long as the economic losses associated with a particular method of care, milking, feeding, or housing are less than the economic benefits, these current production techniques will continue, despite associated animal suffering.

In 1994, the U.S. Food and Drug Administration (FDA) was persuaded by the agrichemical industry to approve the use of an injectable synthetic hormone for dairy production. The FDA seemed to ignore numerous animal welfare issues in making its decision. Bovine Growth Hormone (BGH) can increase milk production an average 10 to 15 percent per cow, further taxing the animals. Records indicate that some BGH-treated cows have produced more than 30 tons of milk in a year. What does this mean in terms of animal suffering? Disease, illness, and infection in dairy cows have escalated as a direct result of increased milk production. As cows continue to be pushed beyond their biological limits, their afflictions, pain, and suffering rise accordingly. The FDA states that BGH can cause sixteen to eighteen additional cases of mastitis in a herd of one hundred cows. Other estimates, as reported in *Livestock Production Science,* suggest that BGH is associated with 15 to 45 percent excess incidence of clinical mastitis. Monsanto, the chemical/biotech corporation that makes the stuff, reports that cows injected with it may suffer from some twenty ailments.

Under natural conditions, a cow could live up to twenty-five years, but on today's modern dairy farms, cows survive only three to five years. As cited in the *Journal of the American Veterinary Medical Association,* over half will be killed before their fourth birthday. This is primarily because of either inadequate reproductive performance or because their milk production levels start to fall. Once a cow's milk production rate ebbs, she will be slaughtered in order to "freshen" the herd. Where does the flesh of a "spent" dairy cow end up? Surprisingly, on America's plates! An article by Joel Bleifuss entitled "How Now Mad Cow?" reveals that Americans eat 2.6 billion pounds of dairy-cow meat annually. The USDA reports that roughly two-thirds of all cattle slaughtered are from dairy stock. And despite the prevailing belief that all burgers are made from steers, according to the USDA's *Economic Opportunities for Dairy Cow Culling Management Options,* about one-fifth of all hamburger eaten in the United States each year is made from culled dairy cows. Vegetarians who drink milk under the misconception that dairy foods have nothing to do with meat production are grievously off target.

FROM GATE TO CRATE: A MOTHER'S LAMENT

> *I took a trip to a stockyard in Pennsylvania and witnessed the beatings of older dairy cows and veal calves. A visual display like that forces one to confront the realities of the system. Being vegan is a matter of being able to look at myself in the mirror every day.*
>
> —MICHAEL GREGER

Dairy cows are mammals and, like all mammals, they naturally produce milk for a period of time after giving birth in order to feed their young. Gestation for cows lasts nine months and, on the average, they lactate for ten months. On today's dairy farms, cows are forced to bear a calf every year in order to maximize milk production and increase profits. Although this is physically taxing in and of itself, the cows' bodies are burdened further by being forced to produce milk during seven months of each of their nine-month pregnancies.

Within just hours after giving birth, a cow's calf will be taken from her. This way, none of her valuable milk will be squandered on her baby, and the mother quickly can be put back into the production line. About half of U.S. dairy operations separate newborn calves from their mothers within six hours, and nearly 90 percent separate them before twenty-four hours, according to the USDA publication "Dairy Health and Health Management." Anyone who has ever witnessed the involuntary withdrawal of a newborn from its mother recognizes the anguish, distress, and woeful cries emitted from both mother and child. By all observations, there is no reason to believe these sorrowful emotions are in any way unique to humans. Cows and their calves wail, bellow, moan, become agitated, despondent, hunt for each other, and exhibit other behaviors indicative of grief whenever they are separated. These behaviors can persist for hours or even days, as Michael Klaper witnessed and vividly recalls:

> The very saddest sound in all my memory was burned into my awareness at age five on my uncle's dairy farm in Wisconsin. A cow had given birth to a beautiful male calf. The mother was allowed to nurse her calf but for a single night. On the second day after birth, my uncle took the calf from the mother and placed him in the veal pen in the barn—only ten yards away, in plain view of the mother. The mother cow could see her infant, smell him, hear him, but could not touch him, comfort him, or nurse him. The heartrending bellows that she poured forth—minute after minute, hour after hour, for five long days—were excruciating to listen to. They are the most poignant and painful auditory memories I carry in my brain.
>
> Since that age, whenever I hear anyone postulate that animals cannot really feel emotions, I need only to replay that

torturous sound in my memory of that mother cow crying her bovine heart out to her infant. Mother's love knows no species barriers, and I believe that all people who are vegans in their hearts and souls know that to be true.

Half the calves born to dairy cows are males who offer no financial incentives to the dairy farmer since they cannot produce milk. Consequently, these youngsters' lives are doomed to whatever grisly end will generate the greatest dollars. Male calves are typically sold for pet food, killed when they are just a few days old to make a cheaper cut of veal used in frozen dinners, raised for beef, or auctioned to producers of formula-fed veal, the ethically worst prospect of all. Essentially, all male calves are considered to be surplus products of the dairy industry. According to an article in *Hoard's Dairyman,* each year the special-fed veal industry purchases between 800,000 and 1 million bull calves from the nation's dairy farmers, representing $120 million to $200 million of income.

On veal farms, male calves are confined in tiny crates to restrict their movement. This prevents their muscles from developing, which keeps their flesh tender. They are fed an iron-deficient diet, which causes diarrhea and anemia in 10 to 25 percent of calves, as reported in a *Journal of Animal Science* article, but it keeps their flesh pale, making it more valuable when the calves are sold for meat. The monetary inducements to retain calves in these dreadful conditions are compelling: *Hoard's Dairyman* notes that there is at least a 20 percent price penalty for veal carcasses not exhibiting the desired light muscle color. During their brief lives, these sweet, sensitive animals will be subjected to near total sensory deprivation and stripped of any measure of joy. Studies at the University of California and Pennsylvania State University found a 3 to 4 percent mortality rate from the time calves arrived at the veal farm until they were received at the processing plant, just fifteen to eighteen weeks later.

My perspective of veganism was most affected by learning that the veal calf is a by-product of dairying, and that in essence there is a slice of veal in every glass of what I had thought was an innocuous white liquid—milk.

—RYNN BERRY

MILKING THE PUBLIC

In order to grasp a share of those consumers who are concerned about health and the environment, and to deflect public sentiment away from the animals, a number of producers advertise their products as being "organic," "free-range," or "hormone-free." Regardless of how a product may be promoted, practically all dairy farms, including those touted as "organic" or "free-range," demand the same abnormal milk production rates of their cows in order to turn a profit. There are no strict guidelines for what is considered free-range, therefore there is no assurance as to how cows at a particular facility are treated. The term is used more as a marketing ploy to generate public approval and higher sales than to convey any tangible level of compassion. Furthermore, lucrative milk production, whether on a small dairy farm or on a large, intensive confinement facility, demands that herds be perpetually impregnated, that male calves be sold for meat or immediate slaughter, and that the cows meet an early and inevitable death.

The dairy industry created the veal market to take financial advantage of an abundant supply of unwanted male calves. It also helps sustain the beef industry with parallel motivation. Dairy cows suffer the entirety of their brief lives enduring illness and pain caused by barbaric confinement practices, rigorous automatic milking systems, endless cycles of pregnancies, artificial inseminations, drugs, hormones, and genetic manipulations, prior to facing the ultimate horror of death, making dairy production certainly as brutal and murderous a trade as meat production. But because the dairy industry is shrouded in civic approval leveraged by a powerful lobbying force, it receives extensive government subsidies, has a stranglehold on our federally funded school lunch programs, and has curried favor within the medical and health-care communities. The blood and tears that go into every glass of milk are masked by manipulative marketing crusades, couched in political pretense, and made virtually invisible to an oblivious and trusting public, making dairy products perhaps even more distasteful to vegans than meat.

> I transitioned from vegetarian to vegan because I came to realize that the same moral motives that kept me vegetarian applied equally to dairy, eggs, and leather.
>
> —CARL V. PHILLIPS

WHICH CAME FIRST?

Veganism acknowledges the intrinsic legitimacy of all life. It recognizes no hierarchy of acceptable suffering among sentient creatures. It is no more acceptable to kill creatures with primitive nervous systems than those with highly developed nervous systems. The value of life to its possessor is the same, whether it be the life of a clam, a crayfish, a carp, a cow, a chicken, or a child.

—STANLEY SAPON

CUCKOO DOODLE DOO

Today's domesticated laying hens are the genetically altered descendants of proud and beautiful jungle fowl from the tropical forests of Southeast Asia, birds that fly among treetops and roost in high places. Anyone who has studied chickens emancipated from industrial constraints is aware of their ostensible longing to reinstate this natural pleasure.

Thirty years ago, the average chicken weighed 2 pounds. Modern farmers, in their zeal to extract as much profit as possible from every captive bird, are now producing a 6-pound chicken in fifty-six days, according to government statistics. As if size were not sufficient, the industry has propagated an interminable supply of birds, making the chicken—not the sparrow, pigeon, or starling—the most common bird on the planet!

In the same way that dairy farmers view cows, egg farmers view hens as laying robots, inanimate machines whose sole purpose is to generate income.

The modern laying hen is commonly believed to be a brainless animal, a sort of black box devoid of the slightest cognitive property. As a result of this attitude, egg workers engender a total disregard for the birds' biological and social needs, are indifferent toward the hens, and bear a thorough disdain for anything they do that might resemble normal, sentient bird behavior. After all, a bird who causes problems becomes an economic liability. Therefore, the industry has implemented standard practices that thwart even the most minute considerations for the birds' well-being if these in any way impinge on profitability. Joan Gussow reported in the *American Journal of Clinical Nutrition* that breeders have actually been attempting to create a hen so genetically altered that she would have no beak, wings, feet, or other "unnecessary" body parts. Incredibly, the idea that laying hens might profitably be bred without appendages irrelevant to their designated role is a notion that has been seriously advanced in animal agriculture for years!

PLUCKING PROFITS FROM PAIN

Paralleling the dairy industry, egg-industry yields have multiplied at astonishing rates due to biogenetics, selective breeding, and brutal factory-style farming methods intended to make profits soar. In 1933, the average yield per hen was 70 eggs a year. A yield of 150 eggs from a 6-pound hen was considered unattainable. Today, a 4-pound hen averages 275 to 300 or more eggs per year. This increase is a result of "advancements" and refinements in genetics, nutrition, and disease control and, in no small measure, industrialization and intensive-confinement systems.

Laying hens are typically housed in stifling confinement buildings where 50,000 to 125,000 birds are crammed into a single warehouse in stacked rows of bare wire cells called battery cages. As reported in *World's Poultry Science Journal*, of the 237 million laying hens in the United States, about 98 percent are kept in cages, and nearly 75 percent have been raised in cages from day one. Revenue, not animal welfare, is the pivotal factor steering industry decisions and practices. At a conference on food-animal well-being, researcher David Fraser established that as the number of birds per cage is increased, productivity per bird is depressed and the mortality rate increases, a clear indication of reduced well-being. Nevertheless, calculations confirm this to be the most profitable, and this opinion is echoed industrywide. It is simply more economical to put a greater number of birds into each cage, accepting lower productivity per bird but greater productivity per cage. In other words, though each hen is less productive when crowded, the operation as a whole makes more money with a high stocking density. The sentiment is that chickens are cheap, cages are expensive.

Although a hen's wingspan is 30 to 32 inches, four to six hens are typically crowded into each 16-inch-wide cage, making it impossible for them to stretch their wings or walk. According to research published in *Poultry Science*, it is generally accepted that the combined effects of confinement and immobility contribute to the fragility of caged layers' bones. Nonetheless, regard for the hens' health and comfort is irrelevant. As reported in the industry journal *Feedstuffs*, nearly half of the layers held in indoor battery cages with five birds per cage suffer from leg abnormalities. Despite associated health problems that can cause severe pain, impairment, and deformity, this type of confinement system persists for the simple reason that it generates a greater financial return.

BREEDING INSANITY

Sound of a Battery Hen

You can tell me: if you come by the
North door, I am in the twelfth pen
on the left-hand side of the third row
from the floor; and in that pen
I am usually the middle one of three.
But even without directions, you'd discover me.
We have the same orange-red comb,
yellow beak and auburn feathers,
but as the door opens and you hear

above the electric fan a kind of
one-word wail, I am the one
who sounds the loudest in my head.

—Courtesy of Karen Davis, adapted from an anonymous poem

The crowding of caged birds has led to a number of significant welfare issues. Hens kept in cages cannot establish normal social relationships, are unable to practice normal behaviors, and have no escape from more aggressive birds. As a result, the system incites cannibalism which, according to Gail Damerow, author of *Chicken Health Handbook,* is one of the most prevalent abnormal behaviors exhibited by chickens held in confinement. Various factors have been implicated as causes of this behavior, including high light intensities, housing systems, group size, nutrition, and hormonal factors. However, chickens kept under similar harsh conditions but who are able to escape do not seem to exhibit the same degree of problems. Cannibalism leads to high rates of mortality in battery-caged chickens, and feather pecking causes injury and loss of thermoregulatory ability.

To reduce cannibalism and other physical damage from stress-induced pecking and fighting resulting from overcrowding, handlers sever portions of the hens' beaks, cutting through bone, cartilage, and delicate soft tissue. This procedure is usually administered without the use of anesthesia, even though it is acknowledged that it is painful and should be done under veterinary supervision so an anesthetic can be used. Recommended instruments for debeaking, as listed in *Chicken Health Handbook,* include livestock disbudding irons, hot guns for gluing, and vehicle cigarette lighters, among others. Beak trimming doesn't decrease the incidence of abnormal behaviors, it only renders the beak less effective in causing injury. For many years, the industry argued that beak trimming was a benign procedure, analogous to cutting nails in humans. However, in *Farm Animal Welfare,* Bernard Rollin relates that it is now clear this is not the case and that trimming causes behavioral and neurophysiological changes indicative of both acute and chronic pain. Furthermore, he states that debeaking causes damaged nerve tissue to develop into extensive painful tumors called neuromas.

Denied from fulfilling normal social patterns and behavioral needs, battery-caged chickens constantly rub against the bare wire of their cages. This causes severe feather loss, bruises, contusions, and abrasions. Moreover, the hens have no choice but to constantly breathe toxic ammonia from decomposing uric acid in the manure pits beneath their cages. The occupational exposure limit to ammonia of 25 parts per million is often surpassed as, according to research published in the *American Industrial Hygiene Association Journal,* the birds are frequently exposed to levels above 50 parts per million. Additionally, an article presented in *World's Poultry Science Journal* disclosed that poultry dust can cause severe lung damage in human workers. Effective January 1, 2009, the use of battery cages for hens used for egg production will be prohibited in the European Union (EU); it's time for North America to join the EU in banning this barbaric practice.

WISH BONES

Intensive egg production also causes laying hens to use more calcium to form eggshells than they can assimilate from food, resulting in severe osteoporosis. Carol V. Gray, professor of molecular and cell biology in the poultry science department at Pennsylvania State University, reported in *Lancaster Farming,* a leading agricultural newspaper, that a hen will use a quantity of calcium for yearly egg production that is greater than her entire skeleton by thirty-fold or more. Consequently, laying hens' brittle, calcium-depleted bones frequently shatter during handling. The results of a study presented in *British Poultry Science* concerning "end of lay" hens revealed that about 30 percent had broken bones upon arriving at the slaughterhouse water bath, but nearly 100 percent had broken bones by the end of processing. Another study reported in *World's Poultry Science Journal* corroborated this research, finding that 30 percent of live birds arriving at slaughterhouses have one or more freshly broken bones caused by the calcium demand for eggshell formation and the restrictions placed upon their physical movement.

If the cost of replacement hens is high, the hens may be compelled to undergo a production process known as forced molting. This sadistic but common egg-industry practice almost always involves restricting water and starving the birds, sometimes up to fourteen days, to shock their systems into another egg-laying cycle. Weight reductions of between 25 and 35 percent are considered essential for an effective molt, even though it is not uncommon for 5 to 10 percent of molted birds to die. This practice is so barbaric that food and water deprivation for more than twenty-four hours was banned in Great Britain by the 1987 Welfare of Battery Hens Regulations; however, it is still legal in the United States.

In a natural environment, hens might live fifteen years, but when egg production drops off around the age of twelve to eighteen months, laying hens are sent to slaughter. According to U.S. Department of Agriculture statistics, the egg industry slaughters on average over 100 million "spent" laying hens per year. Because their bodies are badly bruised, laying hens are considered unsuitable for higher grades of meat. Usually they end up in soup, pot pies, or pet food, where their flesh can be shredded and disguised.

THE PECKING ORDER

Although free-range hens are generally given slightly more space to live in than hens kept in battery cages, there is no industry standard defining how free-range hens must be housed. Consumers generally presume that free-range birds spend most of their day outdoors, with access to sunlight, vegetation, and plenty of space to engage in normal social behavior. However, to most U.S. producers, *free-range* simply means uncaged—with the so-called range consisting of the crowded floor of a warehouse-style building with nest boxes along the walls. Profitability is usually the sole consideration; therefore, the majority of free-range producers try to cram as many birds as possible into the least amount of space. In addition, it is common for free-range layers to be debeaked just like battery-cage layers.

But even if free-range hens were given all the space they could use and an environment in which they could fulfill normal social and behavioral needs, they would still be killed for meat when their egg production wanes, usually after just one or two years. Regardless of whether they were battery-caged or free-range, according to Karen Davis, author of *Prisoned Chickens, Poisoned Eggs,* spent fowl will go to the highest bidder, typically a slaughterhouse, a live poultry market, or an auction. And, like other free-range animals, they are subjected to the horrors of abusive handling and transportation. Hen houses on free-range farms are "depopulated" in similar fashion to conventional factory-style egg farms, whereby farmworkers or contract staff from a slaughterhouse, usually paid by piecework, yank the frightened birds from their cages and pitch them to "catchers," who pack them onto trucks. Even the trip to the slaughterhouse offers no respite from their torment. During transit, the birds are exposed to stifling heat, intensely crowded conditions, restriction of behavior, social disruption, motion, acceleration, jolting stops, impact, vibration, noise, and withdrawal of food and water. And, like all farm animals, free-range hens cannot escape their untimely and inevitable demise.

HATCHED TO DIE

Another problem inherent in all egg production involves the disposal of unwanted chicks. Commercial egg hatcheries are the supply houses for the egg-laying industry. Here, fertilized eggs are incubated and hatched, and the female chicks are sold to replace spent hens. Day-old chicks are divided into two groups based on their sex. Male chicks are of no use to the egg industry because they cannot produce eggs and do not grow large enough to be sold profitably for meat. Like male calves born to dairy cows, male chicks are viewed simply as industry by-products. There is no incentive for producers to spend time and money to euthanize cockerels (male chicks), which they consider to be a liability. Consequently, they are disposed of by the quickest and cheapest methods, most often suffocation, gassing, drowning, or being ground up alive for animal feed. All egg hatcheries commit these atrocities whether they provide hens for factory farms or free-range farms. The USDA report "Chickens and Eggs" sets the death toll at about 200 million male chicks each year.

CRACKING THE MYTH

There are numerous moral and ethical dilemmas presented by commercial egg production and the widespread use of eggs. There is also an inherent incongruity in traditional vegetarian practice, which allows egg and dairy consumption.

Egg and dairy production involve as much cruelty and killing as meat—perhaps even more so. Laying hens endure agonizing years of mechanized environments, behavioral and social manipulation, physical mutilations, intermittent starvation, and brutal handling—all prior to a grueling journey before their final, barbaric slaughter. People who want to eliminate the products of pain and death from their diets should begin no less with eggs and dairy than with meat. When it comes to suffering, the distinction between meat, eggs, and dairy products is undetectable and inconsequential.

INVISIBLE OPPRESSION

My single greatest challenge is to remain centered and loving in an overwhelmingly nonvegan world. In today's world, cruelty and exploitation of other beings—human and non-human alike—are accepted, practiced, and profited from by most every institution of society—from commerce and science to education and entertainment. Unfortunately, the vast majority of Homo sapiens *are either unaware of the cruelty or accept it as unavoidable and even normal.*

—MICHAEL KLAPER

THE LAND OF MILK AND MONEY

Abuse of animals in the animal agribusiness industries is rampant, appreciable, and undeniable. Not so apparent, however, are related forms of human exploitation that exist concurrently.

People who are socially and economically disadvantaged in North America and abroad suffer from many ill effects brought about by the expansion of and dependence on animal agriculture, from limited dietary choices to restricted opportunities in housing and employment. Both the United States government and the public support these practices through legislated injunctions and silent approval of convention, making it difficult for oppressed groups to initiate change in any meaningful way.

Compared with the general population, people of color, immigrants, and women are overrepresented as low-wage labor in the meat-processing and slaughter industries. In fact, these industries are virtually dependent on a steady flow of legal and illegal immigrant labor. As a group, they are exposed to above-average health risks as a result of their employment, squalid living conditions in communities vulnerable to pollution, and environmental contamination from large-scale animal waste runoff.

Because of their precarious social and economic standing, many of the disadvantaged find themselves working in what are considered the most dangerous jobs in North America: laboring on the slaughterhouse kill line or in seafood- and meat-processing plants. Here they are subjected to physically and psychologically grueling conditions resulting in an excessive worker turnover rate and numerous work-related injuries and health problems. Impairments and illnesses commonly suffered from cutting, slitting, gutting, and hanging the bodies of billions of live and dead animals include carpal tunnel syndrome, cumulative trauma disorder, ammonia exposure, tuberculosis (a classic disease of poverty), infections from toxins, puncture wounds and gashes, crippling disabilities, and even death.

The severity of conditions endured by workers in these industries often includes the humiliation of being required to ask for permission to satisfy the most basic of needs, such as going to the bathroom. Those who don't ask are oftentimes threatened with job suspension or firing.

LIFTING THE VEIL

According to research published in *UFCW Action,* a publication of the United Food and Commercial Workers Union, more than 80 percent of slaughterhouse jobs are held by people of color, immigrants, and women between eighteen and twenty-five years of age making five to six dollars per hour. The remainder employed in the meatpacking industry earn six to ten dollars hourly. Industrywide, health-care coverage and other benefits are the exception rather than the rule. Although for immigrants this pay is sometimes twice what they might receive in their country of origin, it is well below the nineteen-dollar rate, including benefits, averaged by the unionized white majority work force prior to the cost-cutting move toward ruralization of animal agribusiness in the 1980s.

The resulting economic reality for the new wave of nonwhite, nonunion laborers is that lower wages and lack of job security leave most of this population financially devastated and vulnerable. It is common knowledge that many workers are forced to leave or are fired from their jobs before any benefit coverage they might receive goes into effect. Due to cutbacks in welfare programs and no protection or representation of a union, workers must rely on their own meager incomes to pay for essential needs and medical care for injuries sustained on the job. Immigrant workers have little knowledge of their rights, speak minimal or no English, are unprotected under U.S. law, and must rely on the hospital as their primary caretaker.

Many women, people of color, ethnic minorities, and immigrants, desperate for work in which their white counterparts are unwilling to engage, have been encouraged and often actively recruited to work in the meat-processing industries. Circumventing organized labor, some of the largest meat-packing firms in the Midwest and South seek out minority and immigrant workers from around the country and across the Mexican border. Standard practices include utilizing labor brokers, employing aggressive advertising tactics, airing television commercials in a variety of foreign languages, meeting with community refugee leaders, posting signs in several languages outside packing and processing plants, offering monetary awards for referrals, extending loans to newcomers, and even working with the U.S. Department of Labor (DOL) under what is known as the H-2A and H-2B Visa Programs. Under these programs, the U.S. government can bring foreign workers into the country if the DOL determines there is a labor shortage in particular industries.

Additionally, many immigrants and workers network within their own communities and thereby assist in perpetuating a constant flow of cheap labor; often bounties are paid when new hires come on board. Once their employment has been secured, their very survival depends on their employers. Fear of reprisal is one reason why many of these workers never report a large number of the estimated thousands of on-the-job injuries that occur each year along with numerous Occupational and Safety Health Organization (OSHA) violations and repeated acts of human degradation.

The thoroughly disempowering structure and pervasively unjust system of the slaughter and packing industries leaves many laborers with few resources to help them leave or challenge their employers. Thought of and treated as inferior, subordinate, unworthy, and expendable, the workers are essentially viewed in the same vein as the very animals they are forced to kill.

ENVIRONMENTAL RACISM

The meat-processing industries generate billions of dollars in revenue and possess considerable political clout, and there is little to deter them from engaging in unfair employment practices and questionable business tactics. Because modern animal agriculture is all about high-density, factory-type production, many communities in close proximity to these operations risk environmental degradation that can jeopardize local residents and further compromise the health and well-being of workers. Serious repercussions include malodorous gases and tainted waste water emitted from packing and processing plants. These have reportedly contaminated drinking water and groundwater around the areas where they are located and have produced ammonia gas, which has been linked to acid rain.

Without the political and economic means to challenge these environmentally destructive practices or relocate to other areas, impoverished people have no choice but to remain where they are. Consequently, poor rural communities have become opportune locations for the slaughter and packing industries to flourish, with little public scrutiny or confrontation. It appears that animal agribusinesses can operate by any means necessary in places where people have been convinced that if these industries left there would be no opportunity at all. Even when millions of gallons of raw animal sewage pour into rivers, threatening water supplies, killing fish and trees, contributing to topsoil erosion, and spreading disease, animal agriculture continues to expand and flourish at the expense of environmental integrity and human rights.

HIDDEN AGENDAS

Animal agribusiness is heavily subsidized and promoted by local and national government officials and politicians who are aggressively lobbied and frequently offered sizable campaign contributions, future employment, or board positions in exchange for industry support. It is not at all uncommon to find former or current government officials as stockholders of or executives working for meat and dairy concerns.

The oppressive tactics employed by the animal-processing industries (detailed in such widely respected publications as *The Wall Street Journal* and *U.S. News & World Report*) underscore the depth of institutionalized discrimination and industrial/environmental racism in the economic arena. They also epitomize the stranglehold that money and power assert over public policy, regardless of human suffering or environmental degradation.

ASSAULT ON THE INNOCENT

> The meat and dairy industries have strong lobbies. They bombard medical schools, dietitians, and both public and private schools with their marketing materials. Then, with the USDA's support and promotion of their products as "nutritional necessities," these powerful lobbies let the federal government conduct their advertising.
>
> —MARCIA PEARSON

Not only are impoverished and vulnerable populations put at risk by working in and living near factory farms and animal-processing plants, they, like the rest of the public, are persuaded by slick advertising campaigns, conventional health-care providers, social-service agencies, the USDA, and other government organizations to consume animal foods and animal by-products. Much of this conditioning begins at an early age through the distribution of nutrition education materials in the classroom. The well-known but now retired Four Food Group model, although developed at the prestigious and well-respected Harvard University Department of Nutrition in 1955, was by and large funded by animal-agriculture industries and their related trade councils and became little more than a campaign to market animal products in all their various forms.

Tragically, the meat and dairy industries' misleading and erroneous nutritional information extends beyond the classroom to the public at large. Billions of dollars' worth of excess fat-laden meat and dairy products are routinely purchased by or donated to the federal school-lunch and surplus-food-distribution programs. The USDA commodity program, for instance, provides meat, poultry, cheese, and eggs to schools without charge. Making matters worse, the National School Lunch Act stipulates that school meals must include a serving of meat or a meat alternative such as cheese or other dairy products. Ironically, a USDA report reveals that school meals have 85 percent more sodium, 50 percent more saturated fat, and 25 percent more fat of all kinds than the amounts recommended for a healthful diet.

While a few school districts are providing more healthful options for students, many are substituting alternative high-fat, high-cholesterol, low-fiber ingredients (such as eggs and cheese) rather than nutritious whole foods (such as fruits, grains, legumes, and vegetables). The implications do not bode well for the millions of youngsters who participate in the school-lunch program, and it is even more tragic for the families who depend on it as the primary source of nutrition for their children. As for the meat and dairy industries, the school-lunch program is an ideal way to ensure future profits and maintain control over the public palate. With their products marketed and disguised as essential foods to those most in need of assistance, there is little possibility that the least educated and informed in our culture will have the access and financial means to explore alternative information sources.

Children and families with low socioeconomic standing are the most vulnerable to nutritional deficiencies and diet-related health problems. Overall, the impact and incidence of ailments frequently associated with diet are astounding. A significant number of both cardiovascular and cancer deaths are diet related. Cardiovascular diseases are the leading cause of death for both men and women in the United States. African-Americans develop earlier and more severe hypertension than Caucasians and therefore have a greater risk of heart disease. In fact, the death rate from cardiovascular diseases is nearly 50 percent higher for African-American men than for Caucasian men and about 67 percent higher for African-American women than for Caucasian women. Cardiovascular diseases also lead all other causes of death for people of Hispanic, Asian, and Native American descent. Moreover—by the government's own assessment—the health of vegetarians is perceived as excellent. Nevertheless, the majority of the people in the United States are being fed a disastrous diet based on animal products whether or not they like or choose it.

The inherent destructive and profit-driven actions of the animal-agriculture industries are epidemic and commanding. Our continued dependence on them and a meat-centered diet blatantly neglects the rights and needs of most of humanity and the natural world around us. One of the most important actions we can take to support oppressed peoples, eliminate widespread cruelty to and slaughter of animals, and restore balance to the Earth and ourselves is to choose a sustainably produced, plant-based vegan diet and lifestyle.

ENVIRONMENT IN CRISIS

If you are not part of the solution, you are part of the problem.

—ANONYMOUS

WHAT'S YOUR BEEF?

The United States of America has often been called the breadbasket of the world. There is much truth to this folklore. For example, Lester Brown, the president of the Worldwatch Institute, a private nonprofit research institute devoted to the analysis of global environmental issues, estimates the United States produces nearly 40 percent of the world's corn crop and supplies over 80 percent of all grain exports. What most people do not realize is that U.S. livestock consume more than six and a half times as much grain as the entire U.S. human population consumes directly. According to the Iowa-based non-profit research group Council for Agricultural Science and Technology, if all this grain was consumed directly by humans, it would nourish five times as many people as it does after it is converted into meat, milk, and eggs. Cornell University agricultural researcher David Pimentel, Ph.D., points out that 72 percent of the cereal grains (wheat, corn, rice, oats, and others) grown in the United States is used for livestock consumption. Only 11 percent is fed directly to humans.

The production of food animals and the consumption of animal products has reached record highs, and no end is in sight. Additionally, the methods by which food animals are raised have changed phenomenally. Agricultural technology, scientific specialization, and industrial pursuit of profit have driven a wedge between humans and the natural world. Most of Western culture, especially in the United States, has marginalized animals, regulating them to commodities and products, tools and pests. This separation from the spirit of life in nature has been nowhere more pronounced than in contemporary animal agriculture.

Modern factory farming is based on the axiom that the natural world and all its inhabitants must be manipulated and controlled to serve human needs. It also promotes the false assumption that technology can overcome any ecological defects and that the environment has an unlimited capacity to supply resources and absorb wastes. Embracing the paradigm of "might makes right," modern farmers view food animals as *less* than human—not worthy of equal consideration—thereby legitimizing oppression of them and making it acceptable to treat them like slaves and machines. As a result, industrial animal agriculture, borne of these self-serving perspectives, has led to flagrantly destructive and ecologically unsustainable methods. Taken as a whole—from irrigation, fertilization, and chemical spraying of animal feed crops to feedlot-waste runoff, meat processing and packaging, and refrigerated transport to the grocery shelf—the process of livestock rearing is the most ecologically damaging segment of the entire U.S. agribusiness industry, and perhaps all other industry as well.

Modern animal agriculture methods can be compared to huge assembly-line factories controlled by just a few powerful conglomerates. The vast majority of U.S. meat products are produced on factory farms. According to the Institute for Food and Development Policy, the three largest slaughterhouse corporations (ConAgra, Cargill, and IBP) control 80 percent of the beef-packing market. In addition, four companies (IBP, ConAgra, Cargill, and Sara Lee) control the bulk of pork production, and another group of four

(Tyson, ConAgra, Gold Kist, and Perdue Farms) controls a near majority of the poultry industry.

Our precious natural resources—land, air, water, plants, and wildlife—are being eroded, depleted, polluted, and killed off at astounding rates. Animal agriculture causes extensive harm to these resources, both directly and indirectly (e.g., pesticide runoff from the production of grains to feed livestock). Nevertheless, few governmental regulations exist, let alone are strictly enforced, that guarantee the protection of the environment and natural wildlife habitats from the abuses of the collective animal agribusiness industries. If our eating habits and methods of food production do not change rapidly and dramatically, the amount of usable land, air, and water and the diversity and quality of all life will be greatly diminished.

THE EROSION OF LIFE

Biologists tell us that there is more biological activity (i.e., microorganisms, bacteria, worms, etc.) below the surface of the land than above. Humans are extremely dependent on soil fertility for food production. The abundance of agriculture chemicals presently used on animal feed crops negatively impacts the activities of these subsoil life forms and adversely affects soil fertility by causing excessive nitrification and carbon-dioxide release, among other damaging processes.

Intensive animal agricultural practices, such as overgrazing, have so degraded the grasslands that soil erosion rates in the United States are now significantly higher than during the crisis years of the 1930s dust-bowl era. Dr. Pimentel's research reveals that about 90 percent of U.S. cropland is losing soil at least thirteen times faster than the sustainable rate. The amount of topsoil lost may take thousands of years to be redeposited. In the United States, nature creates topsoil at a rate of approximately one inch per hundred years. Under less than ideal conditions, as is the case with most western rangeland, it could take several hundred years to produce an inch of soil. Animal agriculture also indirectly affects erosion through feed-crop production and soil compaction.

Environmental damage caused by soil erosion includes but is not limited to the following: sewer siltation, drainage disruption, flooding, eutrophication of waterways, loss of wildlife habitat, and disruption of stream ecology. Erosion can also reduce the capacity of soil to filter carbon dioxide and limit greenhouse gas emissions.

DESERTIFICATION OF LIFE

Without adequate and fertile soil, most plant and animal life declines or even ceases to exist. In *Waste of the West: Public Lands Ranching,* Lynn Jacobs reports that cattle are the greatest cause of the destruction of native vegetation, wildlife, and wildlife habitat, soil, riparian areas, and water sources in the western rangelands of the United States. They are also the primary cause of flooding and desertification, the process by which an area becomes a desert. Livestock grazing has been the major cause of soil erosion on western public lands, which, as a result, are now very arid. Cattle and sheep herds have contributed greatly to the global decline of drylands' ecological productivity (desertification). Overgrazing by livestock has eliminated more plant species in the United States than any other cause. Unable to compete with cattle for available food, many native animals, such as elk, are disappearing from rangelands in large numbers. Other species, such as coyotes, rattlesnakes, and foxes, are routinely killed by ranchers to protect their herds.

Soil compaction, which accelerates erosion and the desertification process, is an extensive problem in overgrazed areas of the West. Cattle, with their enormous weight and cloven hooves, exert an average of 24 pounds per square inch upon the land's surface. Still greater pressure is exerted when cattle are at a run, as in a stampede.

Even when portions of land are set aside as environmentally protected areas, such as national parks, grazing and other destructive practices are regularly allowed by the U.S. government, bowing to pressure from animal agribusiness. A number of national wildlife refuges, national grasslands, and other sensitive tracts are also used for cattle grazing. In addition, almost half of designated wilderness areas in the West are grazed by livestock.

DEFORESTATION AND RAIN-FOREST DESTRUCTION

In the United States, for every acre of trees felled for urban sprawl, about seven acres are cut for grazing or to grow crops for cattle. Woodlands provide crucial habitats for many diverse species of animals, plants, and insects. Research conducted by David Pimentel, Ph.D., indicates that animal agriculture accounts for more than 80 percent of annual world deforestation. Norman Meyers, a zoologist, and other scientists estimate current rates of extinction due to habitat loss to be the most extensive since the vanishing of the dinosaurs.

In addition to depleting vital resources in the United States, the demand for beef has led U.S. interests to expand the scope of environmental destruction to Central America. The United States is the world's largest consumer of Central American beef. Cattle ranching has destroyed more rain forest and caused more loss of biodiversity than any other activity in this part of the world. Tropical rain forests contain more of the world's diversity than any other ecosystem.

COMING CLEAN WITH WATER

Animal agriculture is a major consumer of water resources in the United States. According to Norman Meyers, irrigation, employed mainly for feed crops, uses more than 80 percent of U.S. water, and agriculture in total, as reported by David Pimentel, uses almost 90 percent of freshwater consumed annually in the United States. In contrast, nonindustrial domestic consumption amounts to only about 5 percent of our water, as cited by Betsy Todd in an article entitled "The Effects of Diet on the Environment." Animal agricultural practices are rapidly depleting this country's groundwater stocks. For example, areas of the southern and western United States have faced severe shortages already, and the situation is rapidly deteriorating. Pimentel reports that in the United States, water overdraft exceeds replenishment by approximately 25 percent on average, and in some states, such as Texas, it is as high as 77 percent. The Colorado River has been so depleted by irrigation for animal agriculture in California, Colorado, and Arizona that it no longer flows into Mexico, stopping many miles upstream. The great Ogallala aquifer, which supplies most of the water to the plains states, is overdrafted by about 160 percent of replacement; at this rate, it will become nonproductive in less than forty years, according to Pimentel. There is no technology presently available that enables us to recharge underground reservoirs; therefore the situation is quite grave. Less than 0.1 percent of stored groundwater that is mined by pumping is replaced by rainfall. Irrigated water used for agriculture is often pumped back into rivers after use, causing salinization of waterways from salt leached from agricultural soils. Most summers, the Red River in Texas and Oklahoma is more saline than the oceans. This salinization has a profoundly negative impact on aquatic habitat.

Agriculture is not only the leading consumer of U.S. water, it is also considered by the Environmental Protection Agency (EPA) to be the largest single nonpoint source polluter of water, surpassing all other industries. Fertilizer, pesticide, herbicide, and livestock waste runoffs all severely pollute our nation's waterways. It is estimated that nearly all pesticide applications never reach the target pests but instead widely disperse to contaminate the environment. Crop dusting by planes or helicopters is a common method of pesticide application. Aerial application of pesticides makes it almost impossible to control for wind drift, thereby affecting nontarget areas and species. Drifting also occurs in land applications. Fertilizers and pesticides alone are responsible for more than half of all U.S. water pollution, according to *Gaia: An Atlas of Planet Management*. Since 1945, fertilizer use in the United States has increased at a staggering rate. Nitrate pollution from fertilizer overuse is one of the most serious water-quality problems, along with contamination of groundwater and drinking-water supplies.

ALL THAT EXCREMENT

No matter how you survey it, the United States is knee-deep in manure. The EPA reports that about one-third of all agricultural nonpoint source water pollution is due to animal production operations. A 1997 study issued by the U.S. Senate Agriculture Committee stated that the nation's agricultural officials consider 60 percent of rivers and streams "impaired," with agricultural runoff the largest contributor to that pollution. In fact, feedlots alone are a more prolific and perilous source of river pollution than industrial sources.

Whereas human waste products are required to have treatment facilities, animal waste, which produces many more times the tonnage, has few environmental regulations and no requirement of treatment. Environmental contaminants from factory-style animal farming can include excrement, production water runoff, storm-water runoff, dead animals, dust, silage, bedding, contaminated products, medicines, and chemicals. The EPA rates animal wastes among the top ten sources of pollution. One agricultural textbook, *Modern Livestock and Poultry Production,* estimates that at least 2 billion tons of manure are produced each year on U.S. farms. It further calculates that a cattle feedlot of twelve hundred animals creates as much waste as a city of twenty thousand people. Circle 4 Farms in Milford, Utah—the world's largest hog operation, which produces more than 2.5 million pigs per year—creates more waste than is generated by the entire city of Los Angeles. Other sources set the combined rate of cattle, pig, and poultry waste at around 1.4 billion tons per year—one hundred thirty times more than the U.S. human population.

Factory-farm manure storage facilities are replete with heavy metals, such as copper, nickel, and manganese, because farm animals do not digest all the mineral growth supplements added to their feed. When manure containing these excess metals is spread over a field, permanent soil damage results from the toxicity. Livestock manure that gets into open bodies of water, such as lakes and rivers, overfertilizes algae because of the excess nitrogen and phosphorous found in the excrement. Rapid-growing algae deplete oxygen supplies and suffocate aquatic ecosystems (a process known as eutrophication). The U.S. Senate Agriculture Committee study further revealed that animal wastes are linked to a "dead zone" in the Gulf of Mexico. Algae fed by the runoff has depleted so much oxygen from a seven-thousand-square-mile area of the gulf that it can no longer support most aquatic life. Manure nitrogen also mixes with nitrogen from fertilizers, seeping into the underground water tables as nitrates. Nitrate contamination of drinking water has been associated with a number of serious health problems, including the infamous "blue baby" syndrome. The Senate Agriculture Committee report documented the seepage of nitrates through the soil and into precious groundwater in the San Joaquin Valley of California. This area, home to sixteen hundred dairies, has surpassed Wisconsin as the nation's top milk supplier. According to a ranking member of the committee, livestock waste is an enormous issue for the environment and for agriculture and ought to be a major concern and priority nationwide.

Animal wastes, especially hog wastes, can also contain parasites, bacteria, and viruses, including cholera, chlamydia, and *E. coli*. Outbreaks in the United States of *E. coli* have also been caused several times by meat products and fruits and vegetables contaminated by contact with animal manure. Leaks and spills from lagoons storing livestock wastes have caused unprecedented environmental destruction in recent years by seeping into open waterways and groundwater numerous times in several states. In 1995, a heavy rain caused a lagoon spill of 35 million gallons of animal waste. This waste was three times the volume of oil spilled in the Exxon Valdez disaster and killed 10 million fish in coastal North Carolina. With the combined effects of animal wastes and fertilizers used for animal feed crops, according to a computer-generated model devised by Resources for the Future (an environmental research center in Washington, D.C.), livestock agriculture accounts for almost 40 percent of the nitrogen and 35 percent of the phosphorous that pollute U.S. waterways.

THE SLUDGE HITS THE FAN

In 1967, the Food and Drug Administration withheld approval for using animal manure in animal feed due to environmental, animal-health, and public-safety concerns. By 1975, this policy had been partially reversed in practice. By the late 1970s, municipal sewage sludge treated with waste recovered from nuclear reactors was used as a feed supplement for sheep and cattle. Another environmentally unsafe disposal method developed around the same time was the practice of spreading sludge on farm fields. In 1992, the EPA modified regulations that described sludge as a hazardous waste and reclassified this waste treatment by-product as fertilizer. *The HarperCollins Dictionary of Environmental Science* defines sludge as a viscous, semisolid mixture of bacteria- and virus-laden organic matter, toxic metals, synthetic organic chemicals, and settled solids. U.S. researchers, cited in a Worldwatch Institute report and in the book *Toxic Sludge Is Good for You*, by John Steuber and Sheldon Rampton, report that over sixty thousand toxic substances and chemical compounds can be found in sewage sludge. The Organization for Economic Cooperation and Development explains that sewage sludge applied to agricultural land can lead to heavy metals and toxic accumulations in the soil, as well as salinization and acidification.

GASPING FOR AIR

The majority of hog-industry workers suffer respiratory problems, mostly caused by airborne ammonia and dust particulates in the work environment. Livestock are also adversely affected by air quality in farm confinement buildings. Hogs and other slaughter-industry animals cannot survive well under these toxic conditions without routine doses of antibiotics and other drugs.

Nitrogen from animal manure not only pollutes groundwater but also escapes into the air as gaseous ammonia, a pollutant that contributes to acid rain and other forms of acid deposition. Air contamination also can be caused by numerous agricultural practices such as pesticide use, exhaust from farm equipment, livestock odors, and biomass burning. Toxic releases from animal manure lagoons have been known to create hydrogen-sulfide poisonings in humans and animals.

Global warming is considered by many scientists to be a pressing environmental issue. Not surprisingly, four of the greenhouse gases known to cause global warming are emitted from animal agricultural practices: carbon dioxide, methane, nitrous oxide, and methyl bromide, a chemical used in pesticides. The bromine in methyl bromide is a significantly more efficient ozone-depleting agent than the chlorine in chloroflurocarbons. Agricultural carbon-dioxide emissions occur when organic matter in soil oxidizes as a result of cultivation and wind erosion. Methane is released by animal wastes and biomass burning. Finally, nitrous oxide emissions from agriculture are due to fertilizers, animal urine, waste storage sites, biomass burning, and fossil fuel use. In addition, meat products in transport need to be refrigerated to prevent spoilage. Refrigeration is a significant contributor to the depletion of the ozone layer, which shields the Earth from the sun's rays. Collectively, animal agriculture practices contribute substantially to the global warming trend.

ZAPPING OUR ENERGY

U.S. agriculture uses a disproportionate amount of the total commercial energy available when compared with the yield it produces. At the 1997 annual meeting of the Canadian Society of Animal Science, David Pimentel announced that animal protein production (i.e., meat, eggs, dairy) requires more than eight times as much fossil fuel energy as production of a comparable amount of plant protein. Based on these observations, it is clear that animal agriculture is extremely inefficient and environmentally unsound.

Expansion of agricultural production during the last hundred years has been made possible, to a large extent, by the accelerated use of fossil fuels for the manufacture and operation of farm machinery and for the transporting, processing, and packaging of farm produce. Meat, eggs, and dairy foods require energy-draining refrigeration. Consumers' demand for these products often necessitates transporting them over long distances, further exhausting fossil fuel energy levels.

Energy demands from animal agriculture have escalated as meat consumption has risen; however, feed crop productivity has remained relatively unchanged. Farming is a high-risk and increasingly expensive venture. As prices for agricultural inputs have climbed, the number of farmers has decreased dramatically, but the amount of land and livestock per farmer have increased. Large agribusinesses have moved into states, creating huge factory farms. In order for smaller farms to remain competitive with these corporations, they have had to purchase more land, buy larger machinery, and use more energy inputs such as fertilizer, irrigation, and fossil fuels; these measures cause further damage to the environment, including resource depletion and soil erosion. Calculations by David Pimentel reveal that 10 percent of energy consumption by U.S. agriculture is due to offsetting losses of nutrients and soil productivity from erosion. Because these short-term, narrow-sighted fixes are based on a finite energy source (i.e., fossil fuels), they are a self-perpetuating problem that will continue to grow unless ecologically sound alternatives are implemented.

PROTECTING OUR DIVERSE UNIVERSE

While the agribusiness industries erode our soil, they also erode the genetic diversity of life through hybridization practices of feed-crop seed companies, overgrazing by livestock, and pesticide use. The degradation of natural ecosystems (such as grasslands, riparian areas, watersheds, and forests) and general habitats caused by animal agriculture results in a loss of biodiversity. Runoff from fertilizer applications on animal feed crops can lead to eutrophication, thereby diminishing fish populations. Sediment runoff from overgrazing can decrease the sunlight and oxygen available to aquatic life and also reduce fish populations. According to environmentalist George Wuerthner, livestock grazing has eliminated or severely threatened more plant species in the United States than any other cause. Animal agriculture directly impacts the biological diversity present on agricultural land and indirectly impacts biodiversity through connecting habitats and ecosystems. For example, agricultural water pollutants affect species for many miles downstream from the pollution source point. Domestic livestock, which are all non-native species (except turkeys, which have been so genetically altered that they bear little resemblance to their wild relatives), have had the most severe impact on native biodiversity, including in federally protected areas. George Wuerthner cites many parks in which livestock are damaging federally protected lands. For instance, in one California national park, Channel Islands, cattle have caused nineteen native plant species, five of them extremely rare, to be placed on the endangered species list. In Great Basin Park in Nevada, cattle have significantly damaged riparian areas. At Cades Cove Park, part of Great Smokey Mountain National Park in Tennessee, grazing cattle are compromising the recovery of the red wolf, an endangered species.

In both natural and agricultural ecosystems, many predator and parasite species assist with foliation. In turn, natural enemies help keep in check mites and insects that can be harmful to food crops. The ecological predator-prey insect balance has been adversely affected by pesticide and fungicide usage in many ways, including the following:

1. population outbreaks of pests,
2. chemical imbalances within insects, which adversely alter beneficial behaviors,

3. destruction of many beneficial and natural-enemy insect populations,
4. pesticide resistance in insects, and
5. production of pathogens and unwanted plants, causing farmers to perpetuate the cycle by applying even more pesticides.

Moreover, pesticides and herbicides have been shown to cause birth defects and death in many wild birds either directly through exposure or indirectly by consumption of contaminated insects.

Bees are vital for pollination of many fruits and vegetables. However, most insecticides used in agriculture are toxic to bees, thus reducing pollination of food crops, resulting in massive economic losses per year.

CORPORATIZATION OF ANIMAL AGRICULTURE

Corporate agribusinesses manufacture and market nearly all the food in the United States. Through company mergers and acquisitions, the agribusiness industries, like the rest of the business world, are experiencing rapid vertical and sometimes horizontal integration. It is not unusual for one company to own or have stock in several businesses along the animal-product assembly line, from grain production to animal farming to slaughterhouse processing to packaging to transporting.

These corporate conglomerates consolidate power and secure privileges for influencing public policy and governmental regulation of the industry. Certain animal agriculture corporations have the resources to get around the few environmental laws that exist for regulation of agribusiness. Others simply seek to build large-scale operations in states with fewer or weaker environmental stipulations.

In the past fifty years, the number of farms has declined in the United States by about two-thirds while the amount of farmland has remained nearly the same. Small farming operations have been squeezed out or are forced to compete with large corporations that often have very few ties to and little sense of responsibility for the local community.

SUBSIDIZED DESTRUCTION

The USDA's Emergency Feed Program distributes hundreds of millions of dollars annually to large-scale ranchers. Range management researchers argue that the program actually encourages and rewards ranchers to raise more livestock than the land can handle, which destroys habitat at the expense of the government—meaning the taxpayers. Each year the Bureau of Land Management spends millions of dollars more on range management than it takes in from leasing public lands to ranchers. In 1992, in order to ease the environmental devastation of grazing practices and to recoup a greater portion of tax-subsidized governmental management of grazing lands, Congress proposed a slight fee increase. Due to pressure from agribusiness, the bill did not pass.

CORPORATE GREENWASHING

Agribusiness has a vested interest in making sure that no adverse publicity disparages any of its products. In fact, many states now have what are called *food disparagement laws* that in effect declare that it is illegal for anyone to publicly malign food products by spreading false or damaging information about such supermarket staples as meat. Some critics and legal scholars have argued that the laws, termed "banana bills" by detractors, are unconstitutional because they stifle free-speech protection and serve agribusiness's efforts to extinguish debate about potentially harmful products.

Many national livestock agribusiness groups have vigorously opposed reform and have attempted to keep potentially damaging environmental and health information from becoming public knowledge. Those involved in the animal agriculture industries realize that their practices have come under intense scrutiny and, in response, have resisted outside interference, rallied to maintain minimal regulations, effectively lobbied for protective legislation, and have mounted massive public relations campaigns to sway consumer sentiment and ensure continued profits.

THE FUTURE BEGINS NOW

Being an environmentalist involves more than just recycling newspapers and choosing plastic or paper bags at the supermarket. The overall choices we make every day—whether seemingly minor, like the choice of shampoo we use, or more significant, like riding a bike rather than driving a car or purchasing organic fruits and vegetables—have systematic reverberations for the environment far beyond what is obvious. Individual decisions *do* make a difference. Here are a few measures you can take to ensure your own food safety as well as promote and secure ecological protection, preservation, and balance:

- Know where your food comes from, how it got to you, and how it has been processed.
- Practice veganic gardening—the utilization of organic farming techniques without the use of animal products and animal-based fertilizers. Support local, organic, noncorporate farmers.
- Educate yourself and others about sustainable agriculture and permaculture (an environmental term referring to the development or maintenance of an ecosystem intended to be self-sustaining and which satisfies the living requirements of its inhabitants, especially by the use of renewable resources).
- Confront corporate greed through intelligent voting and selective purchasing.
- Rediscover and reconnect with the natural environment around you.

A vegan lifestyle has profound, far-reaching, and long-lasting beneficial effects on animals, ecology, and the Earth we all share. There are few personal actions that can be as powerful or as productive. What we eat, wear, and do affects the balance of *all* life, not just our own. Can the large-scale adoption of a vegan lifestyle positively impact or reverse the disastrous course of our environmental decline? Indeed, it may be the only action that can.

7

SHOOTING THE MYTHS

And God said, Behold, I have given you every herb-bearing seed, which is upon the face of all the earth, and every tree, in which is the fruit of a tree-yielding seed; to you it shall be for meat.

—Genesis 1:29

CRUELTY BY ANY OTHER NAME HURTS JUST AS MUCH

Everyone realizes that hunting involves killing animals; after all, that's what the whole bloody sport is about. But some people, depending on where they live or were raised, believe that hunting itself is dead—a pastime from another era. I have lived in Pennsylvania most of my life. Here, an autumn walk in the woods is frequently accompanied by the sight of men in blaze orange toting rifles and the hair-raising sound of gunfire in the not-too-far-off distance. (According to the U.S. Fish and Wildlife Service and the U.S. Bureau of the Census, approximately 92 percent of hunters are men.) For those of us who live in or near rural areas, or on the fringes of suburbia where woods have been ravaged, displacing deer and other indigenous species, hunting is not the stuff of legends and lore, it is very much alive and part of modern culture.

Our animal cruelty laws are based on the assumption that animals experience feelings very similar to ours. Anyone who has lived with companion animals knows with certainty that they feel not just physical sensations but also emotions, and that they hold their lives as precious as we hold ours. And why not? The vertebrates—which include mammals, birds, reptiles, amphibians, and fishes—have the same five senses that humans have, a nervous system similar to that of humans, and a brain that is highly developed in the areas that govern physical sensation and emotion. In the same way that only tobacco companies claim that cigarettes are neither addictive nor deadly, only people who try to rationalize cruelty claim that animals cannot suffer.

Even hunters usually concede the sentience of their prey. The most common defense against the charge that hunting is cruel is not that animals cannot feel fear or pain but that the "ethical" hunter does not shoot unless he is sure of a "clean kill" and can "dispatch" his quarry quickly and without suffering. Even if this were true, the simple fact of taking from an animal that which he or she holds most dear—life—would be more than enough reason to denounce hunting as cruel. Hunters who imagine there is no cruelty in a "clean kill" would feel quite differently if they thought the next cleanly killed victim might be themselves or someone close to them.

Whatever our pastime, most people talk a better game than they play. Hunters have the advantage that there are usually no witnesses to their exploits. It is not unreasonable then to suspect that the ethics and marksmanship of many hunters improve perceptibly when they exit the field and enter a discussion.

Nevertheless, even cautious and skilled hunters often do not kill their prey instantly and painlessly. Despite a paucity of reliable statistics, due in large part to the unwillingness of hunters to speak candidly on this embarrassing topic, it is clear that frequent wounding is an integral part of hunting. Studies of duck hunting suggest that for every bird who is "bagged" another is wounded and not retrieved, making for an astounding 50 percent crippling rate. Several studies of archery hunting for deer indicate a wounding rate of 50 percent or more, which hunters concede is higher than the rate for firearms, but how much higher no one knows for sure, or if they do they aren't telling. A wounding rate of 30 percent for all species is probably as good an estimate as can be made and may well be on the low side. Since more than 200 million animals, mainly birds, are killed every year by hunters, this means that another 60 million animals are wounded and left to bleed to death, die of infection or thirst, or starve because they are too weak, too crippled, or in too much pain to feed themselves. There is nothing clean about the way that hunters kill.

Wounding is by no means the full extent of the barbarism of hunting. Some hunting seasons take place while the young are still dependent upon their mothers—for example, squirrel season in many states—leaving uncounted orphaned babies to starve. In the same vein, hunters often widow animals who mate for life, such as geese, foxes, and coyotes, and the surviving mates show signs of grief as heartrending as the grief of any human being.

There is also the terror that hunting strikes in the hearts of the hunted. Far more deer are killed on opening day than at any other time during deer season, and every hunter knows why. Unsuspecting deer, foraging out in the open, are caught off guard when the first gunshots are fired. After the deer realize they are being hunted, they retreat deep into the woods where, in mortal terror, they bed down in thick foliage until after dark. Petrified, they remain in deep cover for days until safety can be assured.

In terms of an animal's ability to suffer, there is no difference between a dog or cat and the wildlife that the hunters stalk, terrorize, and slaughter. The difference lies solely in one's perception. We live in close proximity to our domestic nonhuman friends and get to know them as individuals. Animals in the wild are much further removed from us; therefore we tend to think of them only as part of a faceless herd or flock. This distancing allows the public to excuse the hunter's myth: "As long as the herd remains healthy, the fate of the individual animal doesn't matter." Yet it *does* matter to that individual deer or rabbit or bird, as much as our own fate matters to us or the hunter's fate matters to him. Cruelty is still cruelty, even when it's called hunting.

HUNTING VERSUS HEROISM

Numerous books and magazines devoted to hunting are hymns of self-praise written by hunters who portray themselves as the last exemplars of the glorious virtues of a bygone era. Hunting, they proclaim, instills in its devotees such noble qualities as self-reliance, ruggedness, discipline, and courage. It is characterized as a salutary antidote to the debilitating vices of modern civilization.

This is at best a winsome fable, but in reality an appalling ruse. Contrast the hunters' fiction with the facts. Hunters skulk about the forest in camouflage, wait in ambush for their victims, and kill at long range with overpowering, technological weapons, often going to extraordinary lengths to lure their unsuspecting prey to a violent death. Some deer hunters, for example, hide in tree stands (deer are less likely to notice things above their heads), sprinkle their clothing with commercially available products made from the urine of does (female deer) in heat, and then, in a stratagem known as "the rattle," strike two deer antlers together to simulate the sound of two bucks fighting over a doe, hoping to tempt a curious buck into their sights. Duck hunters hide in shelters disguised as natural growth and place painted wooden models of ducks on the water so that live birds flying nearby will see them, assume that this is a safe place with good food, and descend within range of the shotguns. Duck and turkey hunters use commercially produced instruments known as calls to mimic the voices of the birds and entice them into harm's way, while dove hunters sow fields with sunflower seeds to attract mourning doves to their death.

Equally important is the fact that hunters are rarely in any danger from the animals they hunt. They inflict pain and death on creatures who cannot hurt them. Even animals who could pose a threat, such as bears or cougars, would normally run rather than fight a human being, unless they are cornered or protecting their young. Most of the animals hunted in North America—white-tailed and mule deer, squirrels, rabbits, geese, ducks, and mourning doves—are never dangerous to the hunter. In fact, very few hunting injuries are inflicted by animals; nearly all are caused by carelessness. Most hunters who are killed during the hunt either shoot themselves accidentally or are shot by other hunters. If hunting is considered a dangerous sport, it is not the animals who make it so.

What could be considered so courageous about such an imbalanced pursuit? In essence, hunting makes a mockery of the many virtues hunters claim to represent. Hunters kill innocent, helpless beings who bear them no ill will and whose best defense is blind luck. Hunters entrap and frequently shoot terrified animals in the back as they flee for their lives. Often hunters tempt animals with a false promise of food or a mate, and then kill the trusting creatures who are duped by their bait. These are not the virtues of any era, past or present. They are the vices of bullying and cowardice.

Sadly, hunters are indoctrinated at every turn by hunting groups and state wildlife agencies that are dependent on the billions of dollars that hunters spend every year. Under a barrage of propaganda, most hunters come to believe the rationalizations of the hunting-industry leaders who are constantly forced to defend their sport to the media and a questioning public.

THE COMPASSIONATE HUNTER: KIND BULLET, CRUEL STARVATION

Hunters often say they are motivated by compassion for the animals they kill. Their explanation goes as follows: "Without hunting to thin the herd, the population would outstrip the food supply and, during the winter, the animals would die a slow, painful death from starvation, disease, and hypothermia. A quick death by the bullet is much kinder." Another version of this reasoning holds that without hunting, overpopulating animals would destroy our lawns and gardens and put us all at risk by crashing into cars in frightening numbers. So, by keeping down the population, hunters are "doing us all a service."

These rationales are typically only used for deer hunting and, occasionally in recent years, for nonmigratory Canada geese who have taken up residence on golf courses and cemeteries. No hunters ever seriously claim that they hunt to control overpopulation or forestall starvation among other species. But deer constitute only about 3 percent of the animals killed every year by hunters, making this argument irrelevant to the vast majority of all hunting. Of the more than 200 million animals killed every year by hunters, 50 million are mourning doves and millions more are migratory Canada geese and ducks.

Deer hunters take great pride in "bagging" the largest and strongest animals that they can find, those best able to avoid starvation and disease and survive a cold winter. Consequently, some critics have dubbed sport hunting "evolution in reverse; the survival of the least fit." Without human interference, nature has its own way of reducing starvation. When food is scarce, the rate of conception drops and single births greatly outnumber twins; when food is more plentiful, both the conception rate and the number of multiple births increase.

Like all arguments made in defense of hunting, overpopulation and starvation are unsound. If humans truly believed that killing is an ethical answer to possible starvation, we might apply the same ultimate solution when a human community is threatened with famine. Killing deer to save them from hypothetical starvation is no more ethical than killing humans on the same basis.

But even if we were to concede that killing deer is not the same as killing humans, there is still an air of disingenuousness about the overpopulation argument. Under pressure from hunters, state wildlife agencies—which are, without exception, strongly prohunting—systematically act to *increase* rather than decrease the size of deer herds so that there will be plenty of live targets at which hunters can take aim. This is done through practices such as clearcutting forests to increase the food supply for deer—which in turn increases the size of the herd—and gender manipulation, allowing far more bucks than does to be killed during hunting season. Since deer are polygamous, one buck can impregnate several does, but a doe can become pregnant only once per season. A high doe-to-buck ratio means a high birthrate and a rapidly growing herd. Having deliberately increased the size of the deer herd, state wildlife agencies inform the public that hunting is necessary to control overpopulation, prevent starvation, avert dangerous collisions with cars, and avoid damage to crops and shrubs. Because the agencies' budgets are dependent upon the sale of hunting licenses, a large deer herd means increased sales.

Not content with increasing current wildlife populations, states often import new species with a view to expanding hunting. Elk, bighorn sheep, mountain goats, wild turkeys, and other favorite targets of hunters are currently being introduced into areas where they do not now exist. Furthermore, many state wildlife agencies breed ring-necked pheasants, which are not native to North America, for release at the start of each hunting season.

Epilogue
(In Which the Fantasy Is Real and the Reality Is Fantasy)

"But you don't understand," said the man with the gun
to the doe with the velvety buff coat.
"I will save you from starvation. I will pray for a clean kill
and give thanks to the universe
for the opportunity to shed your blood."
"Thank you, sir," she replied.
"But all the same, I think I would prefer to live."

—Patti Rodgers

HISTORICAL HERESY

Often we hear the claim that hunting is an integral component of rural culture, a time-honored tradition that dates back to pioneer days, colonial days, the Middle Ages, or the Paleolithic Age. In multicultural North America, so the argument runs, respect for the cultural practices of others is a cornerstone of our way of life. It is considered impolite and politically incorrect to attack the cultural heritage of those who hunt.

Had humanity always believed that traditions were sacrosanct, we would still be protecting the abuses of slavery, segregation, child labor, and the oppression of women. These examples are ample proof that not all cultural values deserve preservation. As societies become more enlightened, old traditions subside and new ones emerge to take their place. For our moral compass, we must always look to the future as well as the past. As our culture extends its circle of compassion to include nonhuman animals, hunting and our views toward it should simultaneously evolve. There are many harmless and noninvasive ways to observe and appreciate the animals that live silently among us and in our few remaining woodlands: wildlife photography, bird watching, nature hikes, camping, and orienteering.

In this light, it is important to note that the admirable character traits that hunters often claim are engendered by their sport—an appreciation for the natural world, patience, self-reliance, perseverance, self-esteem from acquiring skills and achieving goals—are derived from the *pursuit,* not from the kill. If hunters carried a camera instead of a gun and photographed rather than shot their quarry, none of the benefits claimed for hunting would be diminished. All that would be lost would be the slaughter of defenseless animals. If, on the other hand, the hunter derives his pleasure from the act of killing, then it is bloodlust pure and simple, and no civilized individual would dare justify a dark passion such as that.

THE CHILDREN'S HOUR

In a variation of the character-building and cultural-tradition themes, we often hear hunting extolled as a way to instill strong values in children. Hunters claim that hunting provides an opportunity for parents to spend quality time with their children, to bond with them, and to pass on the values of the family. It is also argued that an interest in a wholesome activity like hunting can capture children's attention and occupy their time, thereby keeping them out of trouble and away from alcohol, drugs, and assorted other bad influences.

If indeed the beneficial lessons and values to be learned from hunting are derived from the search and not the kill, when parents take their children into the woods to photograph, hike, or camp, they gain quality time and engage the curiosity of the young people no less than if they were killing. Most important, they are not teaching their children the corrosive lessons that (1) concern for the suffering and death of animals is a form of weakness, and (2) killing is fun.

THE ERROR BRED IN THE BONE?

Hunters boast that human beings are predators by nature and that hunting fulfills the essence of what it means to be human. However, only about 5.8 percent of the total United States population bought hunting licenses in 1996, and the hunting population has continually declined since 1975. If humans had a genetic predisposition to hunt, it makes sense that more of us would be shouldering guns every autumn, not less. Furthermore, this opinion ignores the prevalent belief that humans are free moral agents, able to govern our behavior according to our understanding of right and wrong. Few people accept that we are bound by evolution and condemned by our genes to mindlessly repeat neurotic rituals from our prehistoric past.

> *Some say it is natural to kill and therefore it is okay. While it is true that some animals kill other animals in nature, moral philosophy is based on principles, not excused by the lack of morality in others. Some humans assault, rape, or kill other humans, yet we do not condone these actions. Not all other animals act with savagery and amorality; there are many examples of animals acting compassionately. Most of the animals we exploit do not kill other animals. It would seem that if we cannot define our own ethics and are looking elsewhere for models of morality, we would follow the best examples, not seek out the worst.*
>
> —ANNE GREEN

HOLY TERROR

The major Eastern religions have ethical prohibitions against killing animals. Butchering and hunting, for example, are activities forbidden to Buddhists and Jains. Not all schools or individual practitioners may observe these precepts, but they are recognized as ideals to strive for.

In the Western religions, on the other hand, it is often claimed that while we have an ethical obligation to treat animals humanely, God created them to be used by human beings for whatever purposes we choose, and if this causes suffering and death it is morally acceptable because God authorized it. Often used as a defense of sport hunting, this theory is usually tied to Genesis 1:26: "And God said, Let us make man in our image, after our likeness; and let them have dominion over the fish of the sea, and over the fowl of the air, and over the cattle, and over all the earth, and over every creeping thing that creepeth upon the earth."

This verse has been used to justify not only the torture and slaughter of animals but also every kind of environmental rapacity that can be imagined. Any endeavor in which humans participate can become corrupted by human nature and circumstance. Therefore, we have an obligation to constantly examine our behavior against the core tenets of our faith and to correct those that do not measure up. Tested against the ideals of universal love and compassion that are the ethical pinnacles of Judaism, Christianity, and Islam, among others, the notion that God gave us the right to confine, torture, or kill animals for our own purposes fails abysmally. Moreover, the word *dominion* means "authority," and authority is never a waiver of morality or responsibility. Parents have dominion over their children, but this does not give them license to neglect or abuse them. It is our obligation to judge humanity's treatment of nonhuman animals by the same standard. People who use our dominion over animals as an excuse to mistreat and murder them distort this Biblical passage into a claim that might makes right, an assertion that has never been countenanced by any of the world's major religions.

> *Not all religions represent humans as having dominion over other animals, and even among those that do, the notion of dominion should be understood as unselfish guardianship, not selfish power. Many religions teach that all animals, not just humans, have immortal souls. However, even if only humans are immortal, this would only prove that we live forever whereas other animals do not. And this fact (if it is a fact) would increase, not decrease, our obligation to insure that this—the only life other animals have—be as long and as good as possible.*
>
> —TOM REGAN

ANIMALS AND ENTERTAINMENT

The life spark in my eyes is in no way different than the life spark in the eyes of any other sentient being.

—MICHAEL STEPANIAK

HUMANITY'S SHAME

The animal-entertainment and captive-display industries are deeply ingrained in our culture, buoyed by broad public approval and an unspoken sentiment that animals are an expendable commodity to be used in whatever manner humans see fit. As a result, prevalent forms of animal amusement, such as zoos, circuses, marine mammal parks, rodeos, and racetracks, have been able to establish a positive public image that precludes close scrutiny and shields them from disapproval. Behind this armor of acceptance, however, lies a litany of abuse and indifference. Moreover, many are lucrative enterprises that attract tourists, enhance the local economy, and curry favor with elected officials, thereby thwarting objective assessment or investigation.

In addition to the most prominent and more widely accepted animal entertainment industries, there are many ethnic, regionalized, or less conspicuous but equally cruel ways in which animals are exploited to amuse humans. Among the most bizarre or brutal forms are donkey basketball, mule diving, sled-dog racing, suicide races, live-bird shoots, prairie-dog shoots, animal pulling contests, scrambles, rooster pulls, fowl drops, alligator wrestling, bear wrestling, pony swims, bullfighting, cockfighting, and dogfighting.

Whenever animals are used for profit, gambling, or entertainment, it is an open invitation for abuse, whether or not it is overtly apparent. Because vegans consciously avoid all forms of animal exploitation, boycotting these animal attractions is a natural extension of the vegan ethic.

INNOCENT INMATES

Caged Lion in the Zoo
Pacing,
Pacing,
Ever tracing
Misery
On
The savannah
Of your barren cage.

—Ann Cottrell Free,
No Room, Save in the Heart

Dictionary definitions of the words *zoo* and *zoological garden* range from "a collection of living animals usually for public display" to "a garden or park where wild animals are kept for exhibition" to "a parklike area in which live animals are kept in cages or large enclosures for public exhibition." The key words seem to be "a collection of live animals for display or exhibition." But what is the true purpose of a zoo?

Zoos are promoted as educational, research, and preservation centers where children and adults can become enlightened about exotic animals and endangered species. A more accurate perspective is that they are pitiful prisons where inmates serve life sentences with no chance of parole. In her book *Beyond the Bars,* author Virginia McKenna states:

> We would consider it cruel to confine a dog permanently in a kennel. Yet we visit zoos where hundreds of wild animals are kept permanently in the equivalent of a kennel. It is as if we, like the animals, become trapped within the zoo concept, and we cannot see beyond the bars. We forget that wildlife in zoos is still wildlife.

Zoos range in size and quality from traveling roadside menageries to rambling, often dilapidated complexes. This type of zoo is usually located in medium to large cities. Operating losses and cutbacks in funding have made upgrading and modernization nearly impossible. Living conditions for the animals are generally cold, sterile, and problematic, with barren cages serving as home. Roadside menageries and traveling petting zoos are typically mom-and-pop operations. The former may be nothing more than a few unfortunate animals existing on a slab of concrete surrounded by iron bars; the level of care given to these animals ranges from minimal to horrific. From grand openings at convenience stores to community fairs at shopping centers or fire halls, petting zoos are frequently on the bill. Animals forced to travel endure constant stress, often suffering from extremes in temperatures and irregular feeding and watering schedules. Temporary structures used for display purposes often do not provide adequate protection from the hot pavement underneath or enough shade from the glaring sun overhead.

Although many large modern zoos attempt to simulate natural habitats, the result is more appealing to audiences than to the animals. Zoo animals usually come from totally different parts of the world and from very different climates than the cities in which they are kept. Tigers are not native to Pittsburgh, nor are polar bears indigenous to San Diego. Zoos do not enable animals to hunt, mate, socialize, and live as they were intended to; hence, they do little to educate people about their normal behavior.

Most zoo enclosures are extremely small and restrictive. The many animals that naturally live in extended families or large herds are often separated from their group when they are captured and are segregated at the zoo either in solitary confinement or in pairs. The animals lack privacy and have no opportunity for mental stimulation or for fulfilling normal physical, social, and behavioral needs. As a result, most zoo animals exhibit abnormal and self-destructive behavior, known as zoochosis.

Information provided to viewers about the individuals on display is typically limited to listing just the species name, diet, and original homeland. Even the casual observer knows how most children and even adults respond when they pass an animal's cage. Reactions include laughter, pointing, making faces, mocking the animal's voice or movements, and commenting that the animal is dirty, lazy, ugly, stupid, stinky, or worse.

No matter how attractive zoos may appear to visitors, they merely affirm to children and adults that it is acceptable to snatch animals from their natural habitat, cage them, and keep them as unwilling, helpless captives. It doesn't matter if the animals are bored, cramped, lonely, depressed, and far from their real homes, zoos exist solely for the profit and amusement of people. In fact, zookeepers never address what it would take to make the animals happy. This is simply not a subject of expertise. Zookeepers are concerned with creating a good exhibit, keeping the animals docile, or encouraging them to breed.

Preservation research conducted by zoos is generally geared toward improving propagation techniques and maintaining more animals. Logic dictates that if zoos no longer existed, the research wouldn't be needed either. Despite their claims, zoos do very little to protect species from extinction. Most captive animals are not endangered, and natural-habitat release programs are virtually unheard-of. Additionally, if an animal has been bred or reared in captivity, it is nearly impossible to release it into the wild successfully. A report by the World Society for the Protection of Animals revealed that only twelve hundred out of ten thousand zoos worldwide are registered for captive breeding and wildlife conservation. Only 2 percent of the world's threatened or endangered species is registered in breeding programs. Furthermore, zoos are inclined to breed only those animals that are well liked by visitors. Surplus animals and their offspring may be sold to other less successful zoos, breeders, canned-hunt game farms (fenced-in land where pursued animals cannot escape from hunters), research laboratories, or processors of exotic meat and hides. If zoos were truly concerned about the overall welfare of endangered animals, they would be doing everything possible to ensure the preservation of *natural* habitats, not working to create or sustain profit-oriented artificial ones.

Realistically, for the welfare of animals now in captivity, it is better to work toward gradually phasing out existing displays rather than entire facilities. Concerned individuals should not patronize a zoo unless they are serious about implementing changes, have thoroughly educated themselves on the improvements needed at that particular facility, and are actively working to remedy conditions for specific animals held there. Vegan adults and children can learn about exotic animals by observing them in their natural habitat or studying them through films, photographs, and books.

ABUSE UNDER THE BIG TOP

THE CIRCUS IS COMING TO TOWN! the boldly lettered and vividly colored posters shout. Come see death-defying acts, the slapstick antics of the clowns, and brave animal trainers taming wild beasts. The smells, sounds, pageantry, glitter, and romantic facade of the circus have captivated young and old alike for generations. The general public views the circus as fun-filled, educational, and wholesome family-style entertainment. It's hard not to believe this, since outsiders rarely get to see what happens when the show is over.

The realities of this so-called entertainment reveal a litany of cruelty and abuse. It begins when the animals are taken out of their natural habitat and brought into an alien world against their will. They are forced to provide amusement for audiences and profits for the circus. Intelligent, powerful, and highly social animals, such as elephants, and fiercely independent and territorial animals, such as lions, tigers, and bears, are routinely prodded, poked, whipped, and pushed into performing totally unnatural acts. Among these are high-wire walking, jumping through fiery hoops, walking on hind legs, executing headstands, balancing on balls, and riding on motorcycles. There are also instances when extremely dangerous and exploitative situations are intentionally staged to create excitement. Examples of deliberately caused agitation include mixing highly territorial animals, such as lions and tigers; putting together large cats and bears, which are natural enemies; and predator-prey combinations, such as a tiger riding on the back of an elephant.

What do people learn about the different species of animals they are watching? The public doesn't learn about their social patterns or how they live or interact with people, other animals, or even members of their own species. The animals performing in the ring are instead forced to act like animal robots. Basic natural behaviors such as foraging, communicating, and even urinating are discouraged. Circuses demean the animals while teaching our children nothing about their true lives. What the public *does* learn, in particular young people, is that it is acceptable to abuse, degrade, humiliate, and be cruel to animals. This creates a lasting impression, which spills over into everyday life.

The training methods used to break the spirit and control the animals are essentially based on fear, constraint, pain, and food deprivation. The federal Animal Welfare Act does not put any restrictions on this aspect of animal management, so in essence, circus-animal training is a free-for-all. The prevailing attitude is "If it works, then it's acceptable." Commonly employed methods include whipping, electric shock treatment, hitting and beating, chaining the animals for long periods, muzzling, tight collars, drugs, removal of teeth, using the ankus (elephant hook), and martingales (rings with chains attached to the elephant's tusks and to the front legs to restrict head movement). Positive reinforcement is virtually unheard-of.

The general living and transportation conditions the animals are subjected to are frequently deplorable and at best meet only minimum requirements. One aspect affecting the level of care given to the animals is the profitability of each circus. Smaller traveling circuses, known as mud shows, pop up everywhere around the country. The majority of them subsist on shoestring budgets and don't provide even basic necessities, like adequate food and water for drinking, bathing, and cleanup. Neither are the larger, well-known circuses without their faults. The Animal Welfare Act mandates that caged animals have enough room to stand up and turn around, yet even this minimal requirement is often ignored.

Circuses can travel up to fifty weeks per year. Transporting chained or caged animals in railroad boxcars or trucks is particularly brutal. There is no heating in the winter nor cooling in the summer. The animals are frequently forced to spend long periods of time living in filth, with no personal care or attention and little or no food or water, while traveling from one show location to another. Circus cages are designed for ease of transportation only; as homes, they are invariably inadequate.

Circuses contend that the performing animals receive regular exercise and therefore their welfare is superior to that of zoo animals, even though zoo animals may have much larger enclosures. Such exercise, however, is usually limited to cruel rehearsals and stressful performances in the ring amidst glaring lights, unfamiliar odors, and a cacophony of frightening noises.

When the animals have reached the twilight of their careers, either by age or injury, the abuse doesn't end. They may be permanently housed at the circus's winter quarters, often in cages or barn stalls, or sold to zoos, less profitable circuses, private menageries, or even private hunting farms.

The life of circus animals is a truly dreadful and inherently grim existence. They are denied even the most fundamental rights of their natural environment, social contact with members of their own species, and freedom of movement. These magnificent animals are not only treated as slaves, they are further degraded by being forced to perform tricks for human amusement— revealing as much about human character as animal fortitude.

Animal entertainment acts are anachronisms. A number of animal-free circuses featuring human performance artists have arrived on the national and international scene; they prove that animal acts are completely outmoded and unwarranted for the financial success of a circus. These people-only circuses are fun, stimulating, and creative, showcasing the true art of circus by integrating acrobatics, aerial work, balancing, juggling, wire-walking, clowning, dance compositions, and other innovative entertainment. Two of the largest troupes are Cirque du Soleil (Circus of the Sun), from Quebec, Canada, which features performers from around the world, and the Pickle Family Circus, founded in 1974, the first professional human circus in the Western Hemisphere.

TROUBLE JUST BELOW THE SURFACE

Marine mammal parks, like zoos, are another member of the captive menagerie industry. Although promoted as educational and conservation centers where the whole family can learn and have fun, many inconsistencies surface upon closer scrutiny.

The educational aspect is always highly touted by the parks. However, very little, if any, information is disseminated during performances that reflects the natural behavior, habitat, range, social structure, and ecology of the animals. What is demonstrated is aberrant captive conduct, which the audience is led to believe is normal. Even the environment in which the performers are required to live is totally alien.

Whales and dolphins, collectively known as cetaceans, are, like humans, very social animals. In the wild, generally coastal waters or the open sea, they live in loosely to highly structured groups known as pods. Typically, the pods are composed of nuclear and extended family members with whom they interact for prolonged periods of time or for life. For example, orcas (killer whales), the largest members of the dolphin family, live in tightly knit maternal groups consisting of the mother, her adult sons, her adult daughters, and her daughters' offspring, all of whom bond for life. These relationships are so exacting that each pod has its own distinct dialect by which it communicates. Some researchers believe the orca may be the most socially bonded species on the planet. When individual whales or dolphins are captured, the entire social pattern of the group is destroyed. Often members not targeted for capture are either injured or killed in the process. Placing newly acquired specimens in confinement with more seasoned residents results in a totally abnormal and artificial social structure.

While living freely, cetaceans travel anywhere from twenty-five to one hundred miles per day. The sea provides a stimulating environment, with its diversity of flora and fauna and its ever-changing weather patterns, waves, currents, and lighting. In comparison, the marine park's idea of home consists of shallow, concrete, postage-stamp tanks filled with filtered, chlorinated water. The ramifications associated with these living conditions are troubling. Free whales and dolphins are rarely stationary, generally swimming underwater about 80 to 90 percent of the time. In captivity, however, the animals are frequently seen floating motionless at the water's surface. Many experts believe a strong causal relationship exists between this lack of motion and excess surface time and the fact that the majority of captive male orcas, along with many captive female orcas and dolphins, develop partially or totally collapsed dorsal fins. In addition, the harsh chemical composition of the water frequently leads to eye and skin irritations.

The marine-park industry uses the terms *conservation* and *preservation* in its marketing literature to appeal to the nobler ideals of the public. Marine-park experts often describe a captive environment as a haven where the animals can live long lives, safe from the perils of the wild. Following this line of thinking, one would believe that mortality rates would be lower and longevity rates higher for the captive animals. Just the opposite is true. Recent studies point to the conclusion that mortality rates for captive orcas are two to six times higher than for free-swimming orcas. The International Whaling Commission estimates the maximum life span for Pacific orcas to be seventy to eighty years for females and fifty to sixty years for males. Marine parks, on the other hand, state that the maximum longevity of orcas in captivity *or* in the wild is twenty-five to thirty-five years. Since most captive orcas don't live beyond twenty-five years of age, this is a convenient figure for the parks to use. It appears that for this species in particular and for other marine mammals to varying degrees, adapting to a captive lifestyle is not possible. In addition, the success rate of highly touted captive breeding programs is ambiguous, since the parks are not required to report stillbirths and infant mortality rates. Because of these factors, marine parks need to regularly replace those animals who die prematurely. This cycle of capture and imprisonment is responsible for the wanton destruction of complex social structures and callous disregard for the well-being of nontargeted animals. Sound conservation principles are irrelevant when it comes to the parks' turning a profit. For example, the industry has lobbied on its own behalf to keep cetaceans such as orcas and dolphins away from the jurisdiction of the International Whaling Commission. If these species were included, a certain level of protection in the wild would be afforded.

Even if the industry claims of lower mortality rates and longer life were true, these factors would have no bearing on the quality of life for the animals.

Simply put, taking away the core essence of what lets a whale be a whale or a dolphin be a dolphin, just so the animals can live longer for public amusement, is inhumane. These awe-inspiring and magnificent creatures, which possess an almost magical beauty, should never be considered commodities for entertainment. Cetaceans, like all living beings, deserve to live in their natural habitat. All cetaceans should be swimming freely, without human interference.

DOING ANYTHING FOR A BUCK

Many North Americans associate the phrase "the sport of rodeo" with history, nostalgia, and a proud tradition. It conjures up hazy images of hardened and weathered cowboys of the American West enduring countless hardships while taming the land and controlling its beasts. Wide-open spaces and blue skies, working the ranch, cattle drives, and living in the saddle are all part of the sentimental illusion. Saddle breaking horses, herding and roping calves and steers, and branding calves are viewed by the general public as being all in a day's work in the life of an American cowboy. The fantasy of rodeo is that cowboys are merely sharpening essential skills and that animals who are forced to perform are treated like royalty, pampered with the best care and feed in exchange for a few minutes of work each year.

When the actual picture is brought into sharper focus, a startlingly different perspective appears. Rodeo is less a sport and more a profit-oriented big business that dominates and abuses docile livestock to perpetuate its own ends.

There are an estimated five thousand rodeos held annually in the United States. Of these, only about one-third are professionally sanctioned. The largest of the sanctioning organizations is the Professional Rodeo Cowboys Association (PRCA), with a membership of approximately ten thousand. It sponsors some eight hundred events per year with prize money totaling over $22 million. Another organization is the International Professional Rodeo Association (IPRA), with three thousand–plus members. A plethora of corporations—soft drink companies, car and truck manufacturers, breweries, distilled-spirit producers, firearms manufacturers, makers of jeans and boots, tobacco companies—throw their financial support behind the rodeos.

Although the rodeo cowboys have a choice regarding their participation, the unfortunate animals do not. They are provoked to perform and to appear wild by barbaric methods, including bucking straps, electric prods, raking spurs, caustic ointments, pain, and fear. There are six professionally sanctioned PRCA events: bareback horse and bull riding, saddle bronc riding, steer wrestling, and team and calf roping. Other events are frequently added, including chuckwagon races, wild-cow milking, pig scrambles, goat tying, and steer dressing (a team of two or three cowboys on foot attempting to place women's panties over the frantically kicking hind legs of a tethered steer, usually to the accompaniment of crude comments from the rodeo announcer). The list goes on and on.

It is ironic that many rodeo events such as these have little or nothing to do with actual working cowboys. Real cowboys never routinely rode bucking horses bareback, rode wild bulls, wrestled steers, or put flank straps on the animals to make them buck.

The animals who are forced to perform frequently suffer significant injuries and even death. Extensive bruising, neck and back injuries, bone fractures, and internal hemorrhaging are all common occurrences. It wasn't until January 1996 that the PRCA required on-site veterinarians at all its sponsored events. (The IPRA doesn't even have this basic standard.) This rule, however, doesn't guarantee adequate or immediate care. Even if the so-called animal athletes are lucky enough to make it through years of abuse without major injuries requiring euthanasia, the end result is the same. When the animals can no longer perform adequately, they are shipped off to slaughter. Eric Mills, coordinator of Action for Animals, a California-based activist group, and field representative for the Fund for Animals, succinctly explains the philosophy of the rodeo industry:

> Rodeo promoters believe that animals are here for our amusement and entertainment. Consequently, their stress, fear, injury, and death amount to nothing.

The general public must be made aware that every major animal-welfare and animal-rights organization in the United States condemns and abhors rodeos. The following quote from the joint policy statement of the Humane Society of the United States (HSUS) and the American Humane Association

(AHA) reflects the position that rodeos merely advocate the abdication of ethical and moral responsibilities:

> The HSUS and the AHA contend that rodeos are not an accurate or harmless portrayal of ranching skills; rather, they display and encourage an insensitivity to and acceptance of brutal treatment of animals in the name of sport. Such callous disregard of our moral obligations toward other living creatures has a negative impact on society as a whole and on impressionable children in particular. It is, therefore, our mutual policy to oppose all rodeos, to educate the public about our humane objections, and to encourage like-minded individuals and groups to seek the elimination of rodeo cruelties through programs of local activism.

In a letter to Eric Mills, Cesar Chavez, the late president of United Farm Workers, eloquently sums up all that is wrong with the rodeo:

> Kindness and compassion toward all living things is a mark of a civilized society. Conversely, cruelty, whether it is directed against human beings or against animals, is not the exclusive province of any one culture or community of people. Racism, economic deprival, dog fighting and cock fighting, bull fighting and rodeos are cut from the same fabric: violence. Only when we have become nonviolent toward all life will we have learned to live well ourselves.

RACING—YOU BET THERE IS ABUSE!

Many forms of institutionalized animal exploitation, such as zoos, circuses, marine-animal parks, and rodeos, are marketed by promoters in a positive manner. They are described as educational, as preservers of species or cultural heritage, or as fun for the entire family. When it comes to animal racing, however, whether it be horse or greyhound, no such pretenses are employed. Promoters brazenly portray these so-called sports as exciting physical contests between finely conditioned animal athletes. The public is led to believe that all racing animals are well cared for, maybe even pampered, during the span of their racing career, and that retirement for these animals is filled with green pastures, soft bedding, good food, and a well-deserved rest.

The public should be outraged to learn that animals used for racing are actually viewed as disposable and expendable speed machines whose sole purpose is to earn profits for these money-driven industries. If an animal is not winning races, he or she is of no use to anyone. A multitude of abuses begins even before birth, continues while the animals are at their peak, and persists up until the day of death, which is most often early, untimely, and brutal.

Not every animal bred will be a winner. Therefore, selective breeding and overbreeding are routinely employed in an attempt to create the ultimate racer. In turn, these techniques lead to further exploitation and can have deadly results. For example, thoroughbred horses are becoming increasingly fragile. They are selectively bred to be large, powerful animals capable of high speeds, but their legs and ankles are far too thin to adequately support their bulk. Consequently, breakdowns (when horses crumple and fall while racing), hairline fractures, and other injuries are relatively common. Often, various drugs are used to mask or deaden symptoms so that the animals can be kept running while treatment for the actual impairment is withheld. This, along with the fact that two-year-old horses are frequently run before their bone structure is fully developed, leads to widespread premature lameness.

Greyhounds provide another example of exploitative breeding practices. Only about 30 percent of racing greyhounds ever make it to the track; as a result, massive overbreeding is used to ensure that an adequate number of potential racers are available. Since young greyhounds unable to run fast enough are considered a waste product by the industry, each year thousands of them are disposed of at breeding and training farms.

Life at the track as portrayed by the media is a facade of what really takes place. The public sees a small number of elite animals that are the exception rather than the rule. These big-money winners are generally treated well and are usually kept alive for breeding purposes when they can no longer keep up the pace and make money. However, for the majority of dogs and horses, life at the track is grueling, boring, and exploitative, and deplorable living and training conditions are commonplace. For instance, greyhounds are kept in stacked cages for a total of eighteen to twenty-two hours a day. And for many, the only exercise is their thirty-second races, which are run two or three times a week. The dogs are kept muzzled for extended periods of time by some trainers and always while racing or in the turnout pens with other dogs. In addition, racing greyhounds are routinely fed raw "four-D meat"—the meat of diseased, dying, downed, or dead animals deemed unfit by the USDA.

The animals used in the racing industry are literally running for their lives. The equation is simple—speed = wins = money = life for the animals. When a horse or dog can no longer regularly win—whether because of injury, illness, or age—its continued existence cannot be justified by its owners. Horses are rarely given an easy retirement. Most often, they are sold to slaughterhouses to be processed into pet food or glue. Greyhounds face a similar fate. Each year tens of thousands of dogs are slaughtered on-site, sent to be killed at veterinarian offices or animal shelters, or sold or donated to research labs for experimentation.

An informed, caring, and responsive public can do several things to hasten the decline of these already declining industries:

- Boycott and leaflet local tracks.
- Lobby for a ban in the states in which racing is currently legal.
- Write letters to newspapers.
- Work to enforce current legislation.

There are a number of sanctuaries that take in retired racehorses and care for them throughout the remainder of their natural lives. Under the right conditions, some sanctuaries permit individuals to adopt these horses. In the case of greyhounds, there are also numerous national groups that act as clearinghouses to assist concerned people in adopting retired racers.

SCIENCE: FACT, FICTION, OR FANTASY

Most people will agree that it is wrong to sacrifice one human for the "greater good" of others because it would violate her or his right to live. But when it comes to sacrificing animals, the assumption is that human beings have this right to live while animals do not. Yet there is no moral reason to deny animals the same rights that protect individual humans from being sacrificed for the common good.

—ANNE GREEN

WHAT IS VIVISECTION?

The word *vivisection* literally means cutting apart living animals, and in the early part of the twentieth century this was the scope of the definition. However, over time, most people have come to associate vivisection with animal experimentation or animal research. Today it is the generally accepted term for all situations in which animals are used in a laboratory setting, including noninvasive psychology research and dissection.

Millions of animals die annually in experiments conducted in laboratories in the United States and throughout the world. The animals used include common species, such as mice, rats, birds, dogs, cats, monkeys, and farm animals, as well as uncommon species, such as tigers, seals, snakes, antelope, bats, and bears. The specific number of animals used in labs is a subject of heated debate and generates widely divergent opinions.

The vast majority of animals used in research are not required to be counted and receive no legal protection whatsoever. Rats, mice, and birds are excluded from the definition of *animal* in the federal Animal Welfare Act (AWA). Since they are not counted, it is impossible to be 100 percent accurate; however, it is estimated that these species represent between 80 and 90 percent of the 17 million to 100 million animals used in U.S. laboratories each year.

Of the minority of animals remaining to which the AWA does apply, protection is minimal. The act does not prevent even the most outrageous examples of useless, redundant, and cruel mistreatment of animals. As long as someone somewhere is willing to pay for it, the AWA allows any type of experimentation to occur, as described in the following passage:

> Nothing in these rules, regulations, or standards shall affect or interfere with the design, outline, or performance of actual research or experimentation by a research facility as determined by such research facility.

As a result, animals are subjected to a myriad of sadistic and painful procedures, which include burning, mutilation, starvation, electrocution, irradiation, and long-term isolation.

Why Do Scientists Use Animals?

Scientists claim that animals are used because it is the only way they can find the cures to certain human ailments and diseases. They contend that it would be unethical to use untried techniques and drugs on humans who may be harmed by them. Vegans respond to these positions from both a moral and scientific standpoint.

The Moral Issues

From the perspective of the scientist who uses animals for research, the moral argument hinges on the concept that animals are not as valuable as people because they are not as intelligent or that they do not have the capability to reason. However, if we were to follow this argument to its logical conclusion, we would then be able to justify experimentation on mentally disabled people or even infants or young children—something no researcher would condone. How intelligent must one be before experimentation is considered torture or murder?

We do not grant rights to people based on their level of intelligence. Rather, rights are afforded to people based on our empathetic understanding that to deny them rights could potentially cause them great harm or suffering. Why, then, is this not the criteria employed when referring to animals? When confronted with this question, researchers typically reply that "they are *only* animals—they are not human." There is an implied assumption that because animals are unlike us, using them in research is acceptable. Throughout history we have seen the same argument used to justify the exploitation of humans who were unlike those in power, through slavery and sexism, for example. Just as variations in physical attributes and capabilities are not a legitimate moral rationale for the exploitation of other humans, the same standard must be applied to animals. While animals may not be able to function or communicate in ways identical to humans, they are, indeed, sensate beings. In fact, a compelling irony surfaces in vivisectors' logic when *dissimilarities* are used to defend the use of animals in research, while *similarities* are asserted to legitimize its existence.

The Scientific Issues

For more than a century, the majority of scientists have relied on the "scientific necessity" argument to justify animal use in research. For equally as long, some members of the scientific community have criticized the validity of animal research, asserting that it is a flawed methodology.

The number of scientists who question the use of animals has been growing steadily, as demonstrated by the recent birth of organizations such as Engineers and Scientists for Animal Rights, the Physicians Committee for Responsible Medicine, the Medical Research Modernization Committee, Psychologists for the Ethical Treatment of Animals, and the Association of Veterinarians for Animal Rights. These groups of scientists question the relevance and soundness of cross-species extrapolation. While humans are similar in many ways to animals that are used in laboratory experiments, our physiological differences are striking and significant. Even when species closely related to us are used for experiments, the findings may not necessarily be applicable to humans and could potentially have deadly results. For example, although chimpanzees have over 99 percent of the same genetic material as we do, they are not susceptible to many of the diseases that we are and have very dissimilar drug reactions. Therefore, animal experiments can be scientifically misleading.

Because extrapolated data from animal experiments can actually impede medical progress and conceivably endanger human health, a small but growing number of scientists are clamoring for an expanded investigation into alternative methods of scientific inquiry. Alternatives to animal research generally fall into three categories: reduction, refinement, and replacement, also known as "the three Rs." Reduction includes techniques and methodologies that decrease the actual numbers of animals used. Refinement involves lessening the amount of pain or discomfort experienced by animals. Replacement would completely eliminate animal use by developing and employing alternative research methods. This last approach is the one that vegans support.

The push in the scientific community to move toward alternative methodologies has resulted in a dramatic decrease in the numbers of animals used in research. In the last twenty years, there has been a reduction of approximately 50 percent. This is significant not only because of the sheer number of animals that have been saved, but, just as important, this decline has not impeded the advancement of scientific discovery.

PRODUCT TESTING

The most widely publicized area of vivisection has been the use of animals to test the safety of consumer products. There are no reliable statistics on the actual numbers of animals utilized in product safety tests in the United States, since the U.S. government does not mandate researchers to categorize animals by their specific use. However, if declining trends in the United Kingdom, where statistics *are* maintained on animals used in product testing, are comparable to that of the United States, then a reasonable estimate would be 750,000 to 1.25 million animals each year (based on 3 to 5 percent of the conservative overall estimate of 25 million animals used in research for all purposes in the United States).

The number of animals used for product testing has dropped dramatically as a result of public pressure and the wide array of alternatives that have been developed. However, massive numbers of animals continue to be exploited needlessly each year to test new soaps, cosmetics, shampoos, and cleaning products.

There are three primary animal methods by which consumer products are tested: the Draize eye and skin irritancy tests and the Lethal Dose toxicity test. All of these cause trauma, pain, and suffering to the animals upon whom they are administered.

The Tests

The Draize eye and skin irritancy tests subject rabbits, guinea pigs, rats, mice, dogs, and cats to painful exposure to personal-care, household, and cosmetic products. The Draize eye irritancy test attempts to measure tissue damage to the unprotected eyes of rabbits when various substances are directly applied to them. These substances are usually left in the eyes for hours or sometimes days without relief. This level of exposure can lead to bleeding, ulceration, and even blindness. Rabbits are desirable test subjects since they have large eyes and injury is easily observed. However, the validity of these tests is highly questionable, because eye physiology differs between rabbits and humans.

During Draize skin irritancy testing, animals are immobilized while concentrated chemical solutions are applied to shaved and abraded skin. The substances are left on the skin and are often periodically reapplied. Some tests produce severe burning, blistering, and ulceration.

Lethal Dose testing determines the amount of product that is required to kill a percentage of test animals within a specified period of time. The animals are force-fed, forced to inhale, injected with, or otherwise exposed to cosmetics, deodorants, colognes, soaps, and other items until 50 to 100 percent of them are dead. During the tests, animals endure excruciating pain, convulsions, loss of motor function, or severe seizures. Critics point to large differences in the lethal-dose levels required between similar species, such as guinea pigs and hamsters, as an indication that these tests are ambiguous and therefore often invalid.

Consumers are led to believe that they are being protected from toxic products because of animal testing. However, even when animal tests indicate that a product is toxic, this does not preclude it from going to market. The harmful product may simply display a warning label instructing people to contact a physician or poison center if they accidentally ingest the product or if it gets onto the skin or into the eyes.

One of the most frustrating aspects of animal tests is that they are not required by law. Neither of the two governmental agencies that oversee consumer product safety—the Consumer Product Safety Commission (CPSC) and the Food and Drug Administration—mandates animal tests. Certain items, such as pharmaceuticals, are required by the FDA to be tested on animals, but personal-care products and cosmetics are not. The FDA does require that ingredients be proven to be safe; otherwise, the product must display a label stating that safety has not been determined. However, the government does not stipulate that these tests must be conducted on animals.

If the government doesn't require animal tests, why do companies still perform them? Consumer product companies continue to conduct redundant in-house animal tests or contract with outside laboratories, not to protect the public from harm, as they would have us believe, but to protect themselves from lawsuits. If a personal injury lawsuit results from product use, the fact that animal testing was employed could be incorporated into a defense strategy to suggest the company did "all it could" to protect the consumer.

Alternatives to Animal Tests

There are many alternatives to animal testing that can reliably ensure product safety. These range from humans using a prototype under controlled conditions to analyzing the chemical structure of ingredients used in a particular product to determine their toxicity. Currently, hundreds of companies depend exclusively on alternative methods to test their products. Furthermore, a growing number of companies that continue to use animal methods are incorporating alternative techniques into their standard testing regimen.

Consumer demand has been a powerful impetus for the development of most of the alternatives to animal testing presently being used. Market research has revealed a strong reluctance on the part of consumers to purchase or use products that were tested on animals. As a result, a number of manufacturer-funded research programs have been implemented at universities and private laboratories to discover new alternative testing methods and further refine existing ones.

DISSECTION: ROOTS OF OPPRESSION

Each year, millions of students throughout the United States have their first encounter with a laboratory animal. Typically, it is a dead, fully intact, formaldehyde-saturated frog they are expected to cut apart. Dissection, however, also often involves other species, including worms, fish, crustaceans, rats, mice, dogs, cats, and even primates.

In a typical dissection procedure, students slice open the animal and inspect the internal organs as well as the musculoskeletal system. While the majority of students do not question their participation in dissection, an increasing number of students are voicing grave concerns over these teaching methods. They do not want to learn biology—the study of life—through death. The nontraditional views of these students have created polarity between them and conventional science educators.

The traditional science education approach asserts that dissection is an essential component of biology education. It places more importance on the knowledge of the functions of life than on the life itself. Traditional science educators claim that the hands-on experience of dissection—and the subsequent killing of between 2 million to 3 million animals each year in the United States alone—is more important for the common human good than a respect for the lives of the individual animals.

In addition to students, this traditional view has been vigorously challenged by progressive educators who realize that a quality biology education can be acquired while still respecting life. In fact, over the last few years, one of the most contentious issues facing the National Association of Biology Teachers (NABT) has centered on the role of dissection in the classroom and whether an alternative should be provided for dissenting students.

In 1988, the following landmark policy statement was issued by the NABT, to the cheers of enlightened science educators:

> The National Association of Biology Teachers should foster a respect for life and should teach about the interrelationship and interdependency of all living things. Furthermore, they should teach that humans must care for the fragile web of life that exists on this planet. In light of these principles, NABT supports alternatives to dissection and vivisection wherever possible in the biology curricula.

Regrettably, this policy was reversed in 1993 after a small but vocal contingent demanded that a stronger emphasis be placed on dissection rather than alternatives. They voiced the opinion that alternatives were insufficient to train students for careers in the animal sciences and biology.

Currently, only a handful of states provide students with any rights to abstain from dissection. Unfortunately, these laws apply only to students in kindergarten through twelfth grade. In the remainder of states, students can be given a failing grade for refusing to participate in the procedure. The fact that the great majority of states allow teachers to fail students for not participating in dissection sends the chilling messages that a student's conscience is irrelevant and that dissection is still considered an indispensable component of a quality education.

Where Do the Animals Come From?

Animals used for dissection purposes are acquired from a number of sources. Frogs, turtles, fish, and crustaceans are occasionally bred but, because of the low success rate of breeding programs, the vast majority of these animals come from the wild. Approximately one hundred thousand turtles are dissected every year; therefore, the widespread use of these animals could result in serious environmental consequences. As a matter of fact, frog and turtle populations in many parts of the United States have already been decimated. Many herpetologists (scientists who study reptiles and amphibians) believe there is a direct correlation between the decline in frog populations and changes instigated or exacerbated by humans in global climatic patterns, increased ultraviolet radiation, pollution, and habitat destruction. The harvesting of more than 1 million frogs annually for dissection is an added burden that may further compromise the preservation of certain species.

Cats and dogs used in dissection are usually procured by biological supply houses from Class B dealers. These dealers are licensed to collect animals from "random sources." This means they can retrieve animals from pounds, purchase them from the public, or, in some cases, obtain them from "free to good home" ads. It has been documented that some Class B dealers actually abduct dogs and cats or purchase them from illegal or less than reputable sources.

Dismantling Dissection: Compassionate Alternatives

When young people are required to dissect animals under the guise of learning about the wonders of life, we must understand that this shortsighted action can have long-term and serious effects. Exposure to dissection is most students' first direct confrontation with ethical questions regarding the use of animals for human purposes. Rather than fostering a respect for life and encouraging students' empathy toward the death of an animal, teachers who force dissection upon their students choose to promote insensitivity and emotional numbing.

Dissection is the keystone upon which all scientific and medical uses of animals are based. The exploration of the mysteries and complexities of life through the suffering and death of animals has become the scientific paradigm not only in classrooms but also in university, medical, military, and manufacturing laboratories nationwide. Dissection is a first step on the long road of scientific discovery through suffering.

There are hundreds of humane alternatives to dissection. Appropriate and cost-effective options are available for students from elementary school through college. The following list describes just some of the many available choices:

- *Videos and films.* Detailed, real-time visuals exploring the anatomy of humans and animals illustrate the dissection process and the particulars of various species' physiologies.

- *Models.* Newer models are extremely detailed and provide for a thorough examination of the physiology of a variety of species. Some models even duplicate the look and feel of actual specimens.
- *Computer programs.* Computers offer the ability to review and repeat the dissection process in a noninvasive and highly comprehensive manner. Students can learn from their mistakes and thus retain more knowledge.
- *Slides and transparencies.* Detailed photographs of normal and pathological tissues and structures provide teachers with effective visual instructional tools they can present at their own pace.
- A large assortment of dissection alternatives is available on loan to students and educators from the Science Bank, 801 Old York Road, No. 204, Jenkintown, Pennsylvania 19046; 1-800-729-2287 or (215) 887-0816.

As more alternatives are developed and utilized and more students refuse to participate in dissection, a new biology is on the horizon—one which views *all* life as precious, priceless, and indispensable.

BIOTECHNOLOGY: SCIENCE OR BRAVE NEW WORLD?

Many people view vivisection as a morally defensible trade-off between lives. The issue of interspecies transplants most clearly demonstrates the problem of determining morality from a utilitarian algebra of worth where lives are exchanged. When considering the exchange of lives for the "greater good," there are numerous situations where taking the life of one human would save the lives of a number of other humans and thereby lessen the overall suffering of humans. Using equations to determine the morality of actions, it would be acceptable to take the life of one healthy human infant to continue the lives of two other infants in need of organs. Indeed, arguing from the perspective of worth, importance, or priorities, taking the life of one infant to extend the lives of two would be imperative.

—JACK NORRIS

Modern biotechnology has proven a nightmare for animals and has accelerated the objectification of all nonhuman creatures. What was once a science-fiction fantasy is now a frightening reality. Technology has outdistanced our culture's philosophical and social advancements, leaving us unable to use it either sensibly or ethically. This heartless manipulation of animals is now occurring on several fronts.

Of Mice and Men

The first ever patent on an animal was issued in 1988 for the Harvard University "oncomouse," an animal genetically designed to spontaneously develop cancerous tumors. Controversy swirled around the patent process. The center of the oncomouse debate revolved around the ethicalness of creating a new life form that is distinguished by the programmed development of a fatal disease.

Since then, numerous patents have been issued for other mice that spontaneously develop a wide array of maladies. In many cases, these mice do not develop the analogous human disease for which they have been designed. Although their genetic alterations may produce copycat symptoms, the underlying cause is often completely unrelated to the origin of the disease in humans. Knockout mice have had one or more key genes "knocked out." As a result, they suffer from various types of afflictions depending upon which genes have been removed. Jackson Labs, in Bar Harbor, Maine, is the world's largest supplier of knockout mice. The ghastly nicknames chosen for different mouse models reflects a lack of compassion for creatures doomed to a life of suffering based on their genetic structure. "Flaky" is the name given to a type of mouse that develops severe skin problems. "Stargazer" refers to those mice afflicted with an autismlike disorder. Such names indicate a callous disregard for these sensate life forms.

Xenotransplantation: Playing God

Significant media attention has been given to an area of animal biotechnology known as xenotransplantation, the transplanting of organs from one species of animal into another species, specifically transplanting nonhuman organs into humans. Several dozen xenotransplantations have occurred thus far, but as yet not one of the human recipients has survived more than one year. This is primarily attributable to the extreme immunorejection response triggered by placing such a profoundly alien object into the human body.

From an ethical standpoint, it is wholly immoral to breed and slaughter other sensate beings simply to harvest their body parts. There is no conscionable justification for such twisted science. From a practical standpoint, human organs are infinitely preferable to nonhuman organs for transplants. A readily available supply of human organs would eliminate the incentive and justification for continued development of xenotransplantation. The suggestion that xenotransplantation is the most sensible approach to the organ shortage disregards some truly beneficial and significantly more humane solutions.

Although the present system for the collection and distribution of human organs is seriously flawed, it is certainly the most logical point at which to begin to address the problem. Laws in the United States are written with the presumption that people who die would not want their organs to be used in transplants. Those individuals who want to donate organs must carry a card expressly stating their intention. Even if a donor card is found on the deceased, relatives can still countermand his or her wishes. Hospitals have strong legal incentives to contact relatives for approval, thus providing an opportunity for permission to be denied. Given the anguish and trauma experienced by relatives when such approval is sought, it is not surprising that many organs are not procured even from those who intended them to be.

The organ shortage is a social problem, not a mathematical one; therefore, it warrants a social solution. One such approach would be the implementation of presumed consent laws. This means that it would be presumed that a person agrees to the use of her or his organs for transplantation without prior consent. Those who would have an aversion to this arrangement would carry a card denying access to their organs. Similarly tailored laws have been successfully implemented in several European countries. Belgium and Austria experienced an increase of available organs of several hundred percent after the enactment of such laws. Unfortunately, such a strategy has received virtually no consideration in the United States. To ignore such a demonstrably effective approach to the problem could be construed as embarrassingly myopic or appallingly self-interested.

Public education campaigns to encourage organ donations have been conspicuously lacking, and those few that have occurred have been primarily funded by private health charities. The millions of taxpayer dollars spent each year on research addressing immunorejection problems inherent in xenotransplantation, via the National Institutes of Health (NIH) and other federal agencies, have produced virtually zero results. If Europe's accomplishments are a valid indicator of the success of presumed-consent laws, redirecting funds toward educational campaigns for donor organs could provide a quick and cost-effective end to the organ deficit. Regrettably, such a strategy does not appear likely, causing one to wonder if those making funding decisions have some vested interest in maintaining an unnecessary shortage.

Building a Better Frankenstein

Biotechnology is nothing new to the animal agriculture industry. Selective breeding over the course of many generations has produced animals far removed from their natural counterparts. Take, for example, broiler chickens, which are transformed in just a few weeks from a small ball of yellow fluff into such an enormous mass of flesh that their legs can hardly support their body weight. Modern animal agriculture has converged with biotechnology to encourage such unnatural manipulation to take place at an unprecedented high rate. The creation of animals that grow the maximum amount of flesh with the minimum amount of feed in the shortest amount of time has been a primary focus of the biotech industry. While these methods may eventually produce enormous financial payoffs for animal agriculturists, they have only added to the suffering of the animals. In addition, this approach to animal husbandry drastically diminishes a species' genetic diversity, thereby increasing susceptibility to large-scale devastation by a single pathogen.

In a principled society, genetic manipulation of any animal for any reason should raise serious and deep ethical questions. However, genetic manipulation for no purpose other than to allow the animal agriculture industries to realize even greater profits crosses the moral line. It is obscene and should be rejected by our collective moral conscience.

One of the latest products of modern biotechnology is what the industry calls bioreactors or pharm animals. These are animals that have had genetic material coded for certain desired proteins spliced into their own DNA. These proteins are then produced in the milk of the host animals. Nonanimal methods of producing drugs in a similar manner have existed for years, such as splicing the same genetic material into a bacteria, which can then be cultured to produce the drug. Pharm animals simply enable the drug producers to turn a greater profit.

PPL Therapeutics has been one of the leaders in this area and has produced a number of pharm animals, some of whom reveal a strangely twisted irony. For example, PPL developed a genetically modified cow with a gene for the human milk protein alpha-lactalbumin, present in much higher concentrations in human milk than cow's milk. Thus, the genetically modified cow produces milk that is more humanlike than ordinary cow's milk. Considering that cow's milk is not a natural food for humans in the first place, to genetically manipulate cows to make their milk more like ours is truly surreal.

In late 1996, PPL Therapeutics received global attention soon after the birth of one of its products, a sheep named Dolly. Dolly was the first animal cloned from cells taken from an adult mammal. Although the cloning of amphibians had been accomplished years earlier, the commercial applications were much less lucrative. The goal of PPL and other biotech companies is to provide an endless supply of genetically identical animals. Thus, an animal modified to produce a profitable protein, grow at an astounding rate, generate less of an immune response as a result of a xenotransplant, or develop any of a wide array of horrific diseases can be replicated like components on an assembly line.

Biotechnology does not consider the individuality or sentience of animals. They are merely viewed as tools and machines to be patented and manipulated as deemed necessary. Humans have created a frightening technology capable of altering the very essence of life, without first establishing an objective and responsible social and ethical framework from which to make a distinction between what we *can* and what we *should* do. Portentously, humans are in possession of knowledge without wisdom—perhaps the most dangerous combination of all.

Listen with Your Third Ear

Anthropomorphic?
Surely, I am
And
Certainly, indeed,
Are you.
The more the monkey, mouse, chimpanzee
Is like a human being
The more useful it is for you
To cut, inject,
Burn, slowly starve
And always imprison
To watch and study their reactions
To try to apply to man.
But the cry I hear
You hear, too.
For me, a screaming call for mercy
For you a squeaking wheel,
A tool loudly vocalizing
In need of lubrication…

But listen again with your third ear
You don't need the other two.
Listen with the ear of your awakening soul
And you may hear your own voice asking,
What am I to do?

—ANN COTTRELL FREE, *NO ROOM, SAVE IN THE HEART*

THE COMPASSIONATE CONSUMER

I was impelled to become a vegan when I realized that being a lactovegetarian who wore clothes made of wool and shoes made of leather still involved me in animal suffering.

—RYNN BERRY

CONSCIOUS CONSUMERISM

There is an overabundance of merchandise available in North America, so much so that most consumers have become numb and desensitized as to how, where, and from what or whom these products are made. We are accustomed to seeing rows and rows of food in supermarkets and aisle upon aisle of clothing, jewelry, perfume, and cosmetics in discount stores, yet we rarely question the need for all these options. Advertisements bombard us continually, encouraging not only consumption but overconsumption of unnecessary items. Undoubtedly, this is one reason why the United States looks so appealing to outsiders—our plethora of products is packaged and promoted as freedom, prosperity, and power, an irresistibly seductive and tempting lure.

Veganism obliges practitioners to consider their purchases carefully and ascertain from whose back a product was made or taken. Most conventional items and everyday goods are not as innocently made as we might first assume. Experience tells us that whenever capitalism is involved, human greed and demand inevitably open the door for exploitation.

> To those who say that veganism is extreme, I reply that, on the contrary, it is nonvegan lifestyle choices that are extreme. How could choices that cause suffering be anything but extreme when compassionate alternatives are available?
>
> —MARIANNE ROBERTS

EVERYTHING BUT THE MOO

Meat producers like to joke that they make money from every part of a cow "except the moo," and, in fact, the meat industry is largely dependent on the sale of by-products, chiefly for leather, pet food, and gelatin, as well as for sundry other items. Gelatin, in addition to being used in jelled desserts, is a widely used ingredient in commercial baked goods, ice cream, low-fat yogurt, sour cream, salad dressings, confections, marshmallows, juices, pharmaceutical capsules, photographic film, hair and nail products, among many others. Gelatin is made from the collagen of the connective tissues of the sinews, lips, head, knuckles, feet, and bones of cattle. Research published in *Beef Cattle Science* indicates that about half of the U.S. production of gelatin comes from veal calves.

The skin of a cow or steer accounts for roughly 5 to 10 percent of the animal's total value and, according to statistics compiled by the National Cattlemen's Beef Association, about 61 percent of the total by-product value. When a dairy cow's production declines, she will be sent to slaughter, where her flesh will be taken for meat and her skin will be turned into leather. Male calves, who are useless to the dairy industry, are often killed at a very early age. Their fine-grained hides are made into high-priced calfskin used for shoe uppers, jackets, gloves, and wallets. The younger the animal is at the time of slaughter, the smoother and finer the grain structure of the hide and the less likelihood of marring due to scratches, parasite damage, ringworm, dung contamination, and other destructive entities. The most prized skin is obtained from unborn calves—some deliberately aborted, others from slaughtered pregnant cows—which is used to make the softest suede. Thus, an integral part of the economic success of the dairy and cattle industries is directly linked to the leather trade.

The type of meat and related food-animal products (such as cow's milk) that are purchased in North America have a direct effect on the type of hides available for leather manufacturing. The majority of leather produced and sold in the United States is made from the skins of cattle and calves and accounts for most footwear and leather goods. However, leather is also made from the hides of sheep, lambs, goats, kids, pigs, and horses who are slaughtered for meat. Around the world, many other species are hunted and killed specifically for their skins, including zebras, deer, kangaroos, elephants, water buffaloes, tigers, leopards, ostriches, eels, sharks, whales, seals, alligators, crocodiles, and snakes. Although illegal, a large percentage of exotic leathers are from endangered animals that are poached and imported.

Leather must be treated to prevent it from rotting or becoming extremely rigid in the cold or flaccid in the heat, thereby rendering it unusable. Treatments for leather are environmentally unsound; in addition, they preserve (i.e., embalm) the animal's skin and make it incapable of biodegrading. This process has allowed leather artifacts to be maintained in pristine condition for long periods. Leather tanneries not only emit foul odors but also produce a host of pollutants, including lead, zinc, formaldehyde, dyes, and cyanide-based chemicals. Tannery runoff contains these toxic substances as well as large amounts of hair, proteins, salt, sludge, sulfides, and acids, which are discharged into rivers and nearby groundwater. Furthermore, workers in the tannery trades are exposed to carcinogenic substances such as coal tar derivatives, toxic chemicals, and noxious waste.

Purchasing leather goods supports the ongoing contamination of our air, land, and water from tannery toxins. It also promotes an unhealthful and hazardous work environment for humans and contributes to making the rearing and killing of millions of dairy cows, calves, cattle, sheep, and pigs each year an even more profitable concern. The use of leather goods maintains a continual demand that is intrinsically sustained by the food-animal and slaughter industries.

Although the quality and availability of footwear and clothing products derived from petroleum-based materials have improved considerably in recent years, they are, inarguably, environmentally damaging. Options include purchasing a minimum number of shoes made from petroleum-based products and trying to make those you already own last as long as possible. In warmer weather or climates, shoes made of woven hemp, ramie, linen, cotton, or canvas are ideal. You can also find handbags, belts, and wallets made from these natural fibers. In cold or wet weather, look for shoes and boots made from rubber, durable plastic, vinyl, or synthetic leather. Some synthetic shoes and belts are made from recycled materials, so in addition to helping save the lives of innocent animals, they are environmentally prudent.

SHEAR AGONY

Unlike leather and fur, wool is a substance that, in theory, does not require the death of the animal who bears it. Most people believe that shearing is not only harmless but necessary to rid sheep of excess wool foisted on them by nature. Like much information about animal-agriculture practices, this, too, is myth.

The great majority of wool used for clothing in the United States comes from Australia, which produces nearly one-third of the world's supply. Each year, several million frightened, confused sheep are prodded, kicked, or thrown onto large ships, each carrying tens of thousands of the animals for transport to other countries. During trips that may last several weeks, the sheep are forced to live in filthy pens, packed so tightly they can barely move. As a result, thousands of sheep suffocate, are trampled to death, or starve or die of thirst because they cannot reach food or water.

Merinos are the most commonly raised wool-producing sheep. Their unnatural skin folds and excessive coats cause severe heat exhaustion and fly infestations. To reduce fly problems, the sheep are subjected to mulesing, a surgical procedure performed on about 20 percent of Australia's 150 million sheep. A report on sheep husbandry issued by the Australian Government Publishing Service revealed that in New South Wales mulesing takes place in 80 percent of merinos and 45 percent of other breeds. Other provinces reported that 56 to 75 percent of wool-producing sheep were mulesed. Mulesing involves cutting large strips of flesh off the hind legs of four-week-old lambs. Another procedure performed along with mulesing is tail docking, designed to maintain the salable condition of the wool surrounding a sheep's anus, whereby the tail and some skin on each side of the tail stump is cut off with a knife. Because of economic and logistic considerations, these procedures are performed on fully conscious lambs without any analgesic, producing varying degrees of acute pain that may last for hours or even days.

Sheep, like most intensively farmed animals, have been genetically manipulated. Previously, sheep shed their wool naturally. Today's modern sheep, however, produce abnormally excessive amounts of wool. As a result, they are no longer capable of shedding their wool and must be shorn. Sheep shearers are paid by piece rate; the more sheep sheared, the more money they earn. Therefore, speed alone dictates the shearing process. Because there is no incentive to deal with the animals carefully, the sheep are often violently pinned down and roughly handled. As a result, sheep are frequently cut and injured during shearing. Stories of mistreatment and cruelty are rampant among sheep shearers and wool classers (people who grade the quality of the wool).

After being sheared, the animals must endure extreme weather conditions without protection. A closely shorn sheep is more sensitive to cold than a naked human being, since a sheep's normal body temperature is much higher than ours (about 102 degrees F.). During cold weather, hundreds of thousands of sheep die of exposure or freeze to death. The Department of Agriculture of New South Wales pointed to cold exposure as the principal reason for 1 million sheep losses annually in the thirty days following shearing in New South Wales alone. In Australia, lamb losses are estimated at 20 percent; therefore, according to a report issued by the Australian Senate Select Committee on Animal Welfare, up to 1 million sheep are now being protected by plastic "sheep coats" to prevent hypothermia losses. Conversely, in hot weather, freshly shorn sheep suffer painful sunburns.

In the United States, sheep are raised primarily for meat, with lambs being the principal salable product. Due to harsh production and transportation methods, lambs suffer from chronic respiratory diseases, digestive disorders, injuries, and starvation. Industry reports reveal that approximately

20 to 25 percent of lambs die before two months of age. Lamb meat is popular among numerous North American ethnic populations, many of which practice religious slaughter methods that forbid stunning the animals. At ritual slaughter plants, the lambs are fully conscious while being bled to death.

Wool is classified as either *shorn wool,* that which is shorn from the sheep annually, or *pulled wool,* that which is taken from the sheep at the time of slaughter. A very high percentage of wool produced in the United States is pulled wool, making it a direct slaughterhouse product. Because it comprises a minute percentage of North American sheep production profits, U.S. wool is in effect a by-product of the sheep meat industry and directly subsidizes the production and annual slaughter of millions of lambs.

Alternatives to wool include hemp, cotton, ramie, rayon, orlon, and acrylic fibers that can be woven into sweaters, blankets, and carpets. They have many similar characteristics to wool and are superior in a number of respects, including being nonallergenic and easy to clean. Synthetic fleece made from spun polyester is durable, quick drying, and provides warmth without bulk in a variety of rich colors and weights. Some synthetic fleece is produced from recycled materials, making it an ecologically sound investment. Hemp and cotton are very versatile and can be used for lightweight clothing and outerwear as well as for heavier clothing items, such as sweatshirts and sweaters.

Hemp is a hardy, renewable resource that could easily be grown on a large scale in those states that currently rely on tobacco crops for their major income. The strain of cannabis used to grow hemp is not the same as marijuana and will *not* produce euphoria if ingested or smoked. The hemp plant produces high yields of premium-quality fiber that can be used for paper, cloth, plastics, and more. It can be grown on a variety of soils without using pesticides or fertilizer. Replacing tobacco crops with hemp would preserve jobs, save lives, and provide an environmentally sensible product with an abundance of uses.

In general, cotton is not an environmentally sound product because cotton crops are among those most heavily sprayed with toxic herbicides, insecticides, and chemicals. Standard cotton production also involves extensive application of bleaches, dyes, and formaldehyde finishes. Seek out unbleached, organically grown cotton for compassion toward workers and the Earth.

Organic cotton is available in a number of naturally produced colors and a wide array of products, including clothing, bedding, and thermal wear.

HONEY—WHAT'S THE BUZZ?

After the introduction of the British Vegan Society's Manifesto in 1944, a continual debate developed over the use of honey by vegans. The confusion was fully rectified when Arthur Ling, then president of The Vegan Society, published an article on the topic entitled "Ain't So Sweet: The Other Side of Honey" in the spring 1988 issue of *The Vegan* explaining why The Vegan Society does not consider honey ethical. Abstaining from the use of honey is a requirement for full membership in that society, as was stated in its original manifesto, a policy that is consistent with the position of the American Vegan Society since its founding in 1960.

Honey is obtained from bees who consume sucrose-rich flower nectar, retain it in their primary stomach (also called "honey stomach"), and convert it to glucose and fructose. When honeybees return to their hive, they regurgitate nectar back and forth to each other. Then they regurgitate once more and fan the half-digested material with their wings until it becomes viscous, making it more resistant to spoilage. This "bee vomit," the substance we call honey, is then stored in the hollow beeswax cells that comprise the structure of the hive.

Although pollen is the honeybee's primary source of nutrition, honey is its sole food source during cold weather and other times when alternatives are not available, providing precious calories and trace nutrients. Collecting nectar to make honey is an arduous task. During its lifespan, if it manages to avoid assailants outside the hive, a honeybee will have embarked on approximately four hundred trips to gather nectar. Just half an ounce of honey involves between eight hundred and eleven hundred nectar-collecting expeditions.

In keeping with the usual animal agribusiness practice of wresting as much profit as possible from every captive being, many beekeepers have expanded their business to include taking almost every substance found in the hive. In addition to honey, beekeepers harvest beeswax (a primary ingredient in beeswax candles and many "natural" cosmetics), bee pollen, propolis, and royal jelly. Before these materials can be removed from the hive, bees must be forced out of their homes. Common methods used to evacuate bees include smoking or shaking the hives, noxious repellents, and forced air. Even the most careful keeper cannot help but squash or otherwise kill bees (including eggs and larvae) in the process. During unproductive months, some beekeepers poison or starve their bees to death or burn the hive to avoid complex downtime maintenance. The hive may also be burned if bees become infected with contagious diseases. Because excessive inbreeding has resulted in a dearth of genetic diversity, honeybees are highly susceptible to a number of sometimes fatal diseases, many of which are relatively widespread.

Queen bees may be bought individually or sold with an entire colony. Although no genetic engineering has been done on bees, queen bees are typically artificially inseminated and selectively bred for desirable characteristics, such as honey production, size, and gentleness. Exploitative techniques such as wing clipping may be employed in order to keep the queen bee immobilized.

Arthur Ling acknowledged that although the production and consumption of honey may not be among the most exigent issues facing vegans, it should nevertheless be conclusively addressed. In his article "Ain't So Sweet: The Other Side of Honey," Arthur Ling summarized his view:

> It is not intended that [these observations about honey] should deflect readers' attention away from what they consider to be more important, and probably less contentious, aspects of veganism. I also appreciate that the subject must be looked at in proper perspective. I do feel, however, that this is a matter of principle, and one which we should not continue to sweep under the carpet. The Society should give a definite lead to its members.
>
> There is no escaping the harsh reality that many of the methods employed in the commercial production of honey are cruel and repugnant and provide an overwhelming case for ethical vegans to reject the use of this product and its derivatives. To those of us who endeavour to live without cruelty, it is therefore imperative that instead of sitting on the fence, so to speak, on the use of honey, vegans should give the honey industry a resounding "thumbs down."

There are many alternatives to bee-derived products. Substitutes for honey include pure maple syrup, brown rice syrup, sorghum syrup, rice syrup, malt syrup (made from barley, wheat, or rye), molasses, concentrated fruit syrup, sugar, and numerous combinations of these. Candles made from plant wax or paraffin can be used in place of beeswax candles. Additionally, some manufacturers have begun using plant waxes and plant butters (such as cocoa butter and shea butter) in lip balms, soaps, salves, and other personal-care products, making bee products unnecessary and obsolete.

VEGAN VIGILANCE

Numerous commonly used commodities such as fur, down, silk, pearls, angora, mohair, camel hair, shearling, ivory, tortoiseshell, boar bristles, horsehair, animal gut, animal hides, and many others are products of pain or death. Sometimes the connection to an animal source is readily apparent, and sometimes it is covert.

Some people might argue that it is impossible to be totally vegan in today's modern society, and technically they would be right. The use of animal products and by-products is tremendously pervasive. For instance, animal fats are used in the production of steel, rubber, vinyl, and plastics. Hence, cars, buses, and even bicycles are not vegan items. Animal products are used in bricks, plaster, cement, and many home-finishing and insulation materials. They also can be found extensively in everyday products, including over-the-counter and prescription drugs, glue, antifreeze, hydraulic brake fluid, perfume and cologne, videotape, photographic film, tennis rackets, musical instruments, and innumerable other items. Even wine and other alcoholic beverages may be clarified with fish meal or egg whites.

Additionally, in today's extremely competitive, high-stakes global economy, exploitation of production workers is as surreptitious as animal exploitation, and equally as prevalent both domestically and internationally. Therefore, seeking out goods produced by socially responsible companies (and avoiding those that are not) is as important as abstaining from animal products and ingredients.

Vegans acknowledge that purity in an industrial country is not only unattainable but unrealistic, and to maintain the impossible as an objective may very well be counterproductive. Participating in a society that is founded on exploitation places vegans in a continual ethical dilemma. The goal, in effect, becomes trying not to capitalize on, promote, or in any way contribute further to this self-serving, anthropocentric perspective. Vegans are at times inevitably forced to choose between the minutia of ethical consistency and a realistic approach.

I believe that animal industries will eventually be forced by public pressure to divest from all of the other industries they have invaded. Then we will be able to lead a 100 percent pure vegan existence. But until then, I am satisfied with the knowledge that I am doing everything I possibly can to remove products of suffering from my life. If an alternative exists, I do whatever it takes to find it and use it, and if none exists, I go without whenever possible. I have come to realize that, although it is not yet possible in our society to be totally pure in every single way, that impossibility does not negate the significance of the honest attempt to live a purely vegan life. That attempt, in itself, sets a truly important example of nonviolence and leads the way to a better world.

—SHARI KALINA

The vegan aim should not be for perfection, as this places undue emphasis on that which cannot, at present, be achieved and undoubtedly will lead to disappointment. In actuality, it is the sincere and steadfast journey itself that becomes the destination. Admittedly, it is unrealistic to believe that the world will become vegan in most of our lifetimes; however, this should in no way deter anyone from trying. As Margaret Mead said, "Never doubt that a small group of thoughtful, committed citizens can change the world; indeed, it's the only thing that ever has." The honorable, admirable, and achievable vegan mission is to ceaselessly strive to do one's best. This simple charge is more than enough to keep most vegans (and nonvegans, too) challenged, focused, and on task.

THE BODY BEAUTIFUL

BEAUTY AT WHAT COST?

The term *cruelty-free* was coined in the 1950s by the late Muriel, Lady Dowding, wife of Hugh, Lord Dowding, who was known as an antivivisectionist and advocate of animal rights in the House of Lords. Appalled by the wearing of furs by "otherwise kind and gentle women," Lady Dowding was compelled to make them understand the cruelty inherent in this barbaric trade. She decided to try to persuade firms that made simulated fur coats to advertise that their garments had caused no suffering. She thought that attaching a label to this effect would make some people stop and think and realize the cruelty involved in making real furs. After numerous rejections, one firm finally agreed to cooperate. Three weeks later, little labels bearing the slogan "Beauty Without Cruelty" were sewn into some coats. Several influential women in London society were drawn to the idea. They, along with Lady

Dowding, formed a volunteer committee to help spread the cruelty-free concept through fashion shows featuring simulated furs. Their first show was a surprisingly huge success and led to subsequent events in London and other large cities in England.

Lady Dowding soon ventured into other areas of the fashion business, exploring and exposing the brutality inflicted on animals in the clothing, toiletries, and cosmetics industries. In 1959, she founded the nonprofit charitable organization Beauty Without Cruelty, and eventually established several international branches in Australia, New Zealand, the United States, South Africa, and India.

Outraged by her discovery of the animal ingredients and testing routinely involved in producing commercial toiletries and cosmetics, Lady Dowding pioneered Beauty Without Cruelty Cosmetics in 1963, which later became a company independent of the nonprofit group. The new product line was not tested on animals and included no direct slaughter ingredients, although some items contained animal by-products such as lanolin and beeswax. (Today, all Beauty Without Cruelty products are entirely vegan.) When the products were not well received by stores, Lady Dowding opened the first Beauty Without Cruelty Boutique in London in the mid-1960s. Well-known fashion models and designers helped raise the profile of Beauty Without Cruelty and broadened its international appeal.

BUYER BEWARE

In 1972, Beauty Without Cruelty (BWC) USA was formed by Ethel Thurston (chair of the organization), Virginia Milliken, and Gretchen Wyler, under the guiding hand of Lady Dowding. Shortly thereafter, BWC USA began publishing its pioneering guide to cruelty-free cosmetic companies. In 1977, Thurston, Milliken, and Wyler helped found the American Fund for Alternatives to Animal Research (AFAAR) to finance the development of nonanimal tests. Among their scientific advisers were distinguished leaders in the field of alternative testing including John Petricciani, Ph.D., Roland Nardone, Ph.D., and Joseph Leighton, Ph.D.

In the early 1970s, Marcia Pearson, then a professional fashion model and founder of the West Coast–based Fashion With Compassion, a group that presents fashion shows featuring American-made clothing woven from plant and synthetic fibers, corresponded with Lady Dowding and received some of her Beauty Without Cruelty brochures. Through her public appearances, her work in the fashion industry, and networking with other concerned groups, Marcia Pearson, along with other animal activists, helped popularize the term *cruelty-free* and introduced it to U.S. audiences. It quickly became a buzz word of the animal-rights and vegetarian movements in the late seventies and eighties and captured the attention and imagination of an incredulous public. Around the same time, a spirited campaign against the Draize eye irritancy test conducted on rabbits by cosmetic companies was launched by Henry Spira. It had a far-reaching impact. The concept that such experiments were unnecessary, combined with the dichotomy of an industry both devoted to beauty and deeply involved in the suffering and torture of animals, proved to be a powerful stimulus for change. Interestingly, the "natural" products industry concurrently discovered that putting a "cruelty-free" label on merchandise could be an effective way to invite consumer confidence and loyalty and therefore generate higher revenues.

In its purest sense, the term *cruelty-free* means ethically produced: (1) Neither the individual ingredients nor the finished product have been tested on animals, and (2) the product is 100 percent free of animal-derived ingredients. Some manufacturers have used the term *cruelty-free* to indicate that compounded products, not necessarily their individual components, have not been tested on animals. Furthermore, these products may still contain animal-derived ingredients. If so-called cruelty-free items can still contain animal-tested ingredients and/or animal products or by-products, what authority and clarity does the term actually have? For the consumer, the cruelty-free label has become muddled, misconstrued, and somewhat meaningless. In England, the birthplace of the vegan movement, the term *cruelty-free* is no longer commonly used on packaging because of its ambiguity. According to The British Vegan Society, confusion often arose because the term sometimes meant "not tested on animals" while the product still contained cruelly obtained animal ingredients. Manufacturers in England are now inclined to use the term *animal-free* to mean free of animal testing *and* ingredients. The Vegan Society considers *animal-free* to be a more accurate term that allows vegans to make humane and informed choices.

SEARCHING FOR SOLUTIONS

Product labels can be baffling. Some ingredients, such as glycerin and stearates, can be derived from either vegetable or animal sources, and manufacturers typically do not specify an ingredient's origin. Some labels list ingredients that are ten syllables long and require an advanced degree in chemistry to interpret accurately. Author, teacher, vegetarian historian, and fourteen-year vegan Rynn Berry recognizes the inescapable intrusion of animal suffering:

> A difficult challenge I've faced being vegan is simply trying to live a cruelty-free life in a society in which practically every commercial product is polluted with animal ingredients and animal pain.

Several animal-rights groups and vegan organizations periodically publish listings that specify those companies still utilizing animal tests, those that have stopped animal testing, and those that have never conducted animal tests. These publications may also list vegan companies and/or product lines that the manufacturers claim are vegan, items that the manufacturers say do not contain animal products but may contain animal by-products (e.g., lanolin, beeswax, propolis, honey, whey, etc.) and items that are animal based. Although these lists are extremely helpful, all information is provided by the companies and is not verified by an outside source.

What some manufacturers consider vegan and what practicing vegans consider vegan may differ radically. There are products labeled "vegan" and "cruelty-free" that contain honey, lanolin, whey, or other nonvegan ingredients. Herein lies the problem with manufacturers' evaluating their own products. When a seal, symbol, or designation becomes financially rewarding and thus self-serving, how can there be objectivity if the process for determining compliance is self-enforced and self-regulated by the very industries that stand to profit the most?

For now, it is best to read product labels carefully, even if some sort of cruelty-free seal is on the package. Many companies, in a rush to capitalize on public sentiment, have designed their own logos or incorporated logos from humane or animal-rights organizations that have honorable intentions but no ability to substantiate a company's claims. A walk through any natural-products store reveals nearly as many different symbols and slogans as there are products. This does not imply that manufacturers are conducting business unethically; however, without outside verification, there is simply no way to guarantee that a company's statements are fact.

Look for hidden animal ingredients in products and contact manufacturers personally if you have any questions. Many manufacturers have toll-free numbers direct to their customer service departments. Be forewarned, however, that the term *vegan* is still foreign to many manufacturers, and you may be called upon to educate customer service representatives about its meaning. It is important to let the natural-products industry know that an item could hardly be considered cruelty-free if, instead of being *tested* on animals, it *contains* them. Until manufacturers believe there is a strong consumer demand for truly animal-free products—those with no animal testing of individual ingredients as well as of compounded finished products *and* no animal ingredients of any kind—and this becomes the prevailing standard industrywide, there will continue to be confusion, misrepresentation, and an unseemly void in the marketplace.

12

ETHICS IN ACTION

To the greatest extent possible, I try to make choices that involve the least amount of cruelty and environmental damage. I am interested in sustainable agriculture, environmental issues, human rights, and my interconnectedness in the web of all life. It is a great pleasure for me to find products and practices that have a positive effect on living beings and the environment, rather than a negative one.

—Vesanto Melina

BEYOND DIET AND CLOTHING

Embracing veganism compels practitioners to live moral and compassionate lives while minimizing their impact on the Earth and its resources. The American Vegan Society's tenet of "dynamic harmlessness," doing the least harm and the most good, encourages vegans to search for options that will protect and improve the lives of all living beings as well as eliminate suffering, bring about the responsible use of natural resources, and inspire peace and harmony among people. Consequently, veganism is not passive self-denial. On the contrary, it instills active and vibrant responsibility for initiating positive social change by presenting a constant challenge to consistently seek out the highest ideal.

It is as if my eyes have been opened for the first time to the many gifts present in life. I feel challenged to live by the inner wisdom of my spirit and the voice within my heart. I'm finding that because I am mindful of my actions, right down to reading labels, shopping for organic foods, and riding a bicycle instead of driving and owning a car, my life is actually simpler and more meaningful than when I drove an Alpha Romeo and wore silk suits. It's a path that has increased my choices because I take the time to remind myself of what's truly beautiful rather than feeling divided and overwhelmed and like the world "out there" is someone else's problem and it has nothing to do with me, my thoughts, or my actions.

—Mae Lee Sun

Because the vegan ethic encompasses every area of life, there are many facets of daily living that nonvegans may take for granted but which vegans must carefully consider. When an individual chooses veganism, she or he quickly discovers a multitude of unanticipated challenges. The following are just a few examples.

OCCUPATIONAL CHOICES

After people have been vegan for a while, they sometimes begin assessing their lives to see how they could be of greater service to others or feel more purposeful. Oftentimes, this leads to a reevaluation of what they are doing for a living. Certain jobs, such as dairy farmer, vivisector, or butcher, are blatantly incompatible with vegan principles. Others, such as working as a server in a steakhouse, selling leather footwear in a shoe store, or being employed in a pet shop, are more subtly contradictory.

Switching careers is hard, and at times it seems easier to bend the ethical rules than to start job hunting, go back to school, or get retrained. Yet, when individuals are conflicted between their ethics and their livelihood, it becomes exceptionally draining. There is a constant need to justify to yourself and to others why the work you are doing should be considered acceptable, while in your heart you know it is not. Rationalizing is unquestionably time consuming, unproductive, and exhausting. By the time people realize the mental effort they are expending, they naturally come to the conclusion that aligning their occupational choice with their ethics is the only reasonable alternative.

Many vegans want to do more than simply maintain the status quo. Consequently, they may supplement their day jobs with activist work on behalf of people, animals, or the environment. By day, Kevin Pickard works as a computer programmer and analyst. But in his spare time, Kevin has served as president of the Toronto Vegetarian Society (the largest vegetarian society in North America), vice president of the Vegetarian Union of North America, and as a council member for the International Vegetarian Union. About his work, Kevin says:

> My full-time job puts the veggies on my plate, so to speak, but
> I see my volunteer work as my real job.

Saurabh Dalal's life is another example of incredible yet widely pervasive vegan commitment and passion. Saurabh holds master-of-science degrees in electrical engineering and applied physics, is completing coursework for his Ph.D., and is employed as an optical engineer and physicist. Despite these grueling demands, Saurabh has served as president of the Vegetarian Society of Washington, D.C. (the oldest vegetarian society in North America), secretary of the Vegetarian Union of North America, honorary regional secretary for North America for the International Vegetarian Union, and has coordinated a variety of select projects for a number of other vegetarian organizations and religious groups.

Some vegans find their volunteer work so satisfying that they decide to pursue it as a vocation. Some people are compelled to disband their often lucrative professions and seek work that advances the vegan cause, as did Marianne Roberts, who graduated Phi Beta Kappa from Vassar College and holds a master of business administration from Harvard University:

> I have been haunted for years by a very graphic photograph of
> a beagle burned in a vivisection experiment. It was absolutely gut
> wrenching! I couldn't get it out of my mind for several months.
> Finally, I was so tormented that I quit my job and went to work
> for an animal-rights organization.

Shelton Walden has a bachelor of arts in political science from Fordham University and is currently a graduate student at Rutgers University in environmental and medical history. As the host and producer of the weekly radio show *Walden's Pond,* broadcast from New York City, which focuses on animal rights, human rights, health, veganism, and the environment, Shelton epitomizes the desire and quest for constructive vegan work:

> Being a vegan contributed to my unique career perspective. Had I not become a vegan, my radio program would not have the focus it has, and I would not be aware of how animal exploitation affects every minute aspect of our lives. Veganism has helped me understand the fragility of all life and the necessity for us to respect the integrity of all life-forms.

As her vegan awareness grew, Yale-educated Hillary Morris experienced a series of revelations during her short career in the ruthless field of high finance:

> I worked on Wall Street as a financial analyst for two years. I could have stayed longer. I could have earned a fat salary brokering deals for huge multinationals. Except for one thing. During my employment there, I became a vegan. Perhaps it was in response to the morally corrupt industry in which I was working—I felt a need to reconnect with something truly good, truly selfless. In any case, when I became a vegan while working in that environment, I began to notice things that up until that point my consciousness was unable to see: the connection between my work financing an oil refinery and the degradation of the Earth's environment; the connection between working on a deal to finance mining and exploration in a remote and occupied portion of Indonesia and the suffering of indigenous cultures. In short, I began to realize the connection between my work, my life, and the state of the world. I began to realize that all things are connected and that everything I did had repercussions not only for myself and the ones around me, but around the world.
>
> The last straw came when I was asked to work on a deal to finance a chicken processing factory. I finally realized that I needed to do work that was holistically sound and complete. So

I left Wall Street and began studying traditional Chinese medicine and learning about holistic ways of healing. I am rediscovering not only my connection to the Earth and to animals but also to my own self—who I am, what I desire in life, and what sort of legacy I wish to leave for the Earth's children. I know other people can do this—if they follow their hearts and have faith, everything they ever dreamed will come true.

Physician and author Michael Klaper found that after adopting a vegan lifestyle he was left with no other option than to make the extension of his compassionate ethic part of his life's work and mission:

To watch the beauty of the natural world desecrated and to witness the death and destruction of sentient beings caused by human greed and the lust for power has been excruciating—and grows more so daily. To create increased awareness of the benefits of a vegan diet and lifestyle in today's flesh-addicted, flesh-indulgent global society is a formidable task. I would gladly swap with Hercules for a run at the Augean Stables. Yet, helping to create a more vegan world is the most noble task of which I can conceive and one certainly worthy as a life goal. At this point, there is nothing else for me to do.

Of course, becoming vegan doesn't always necessitate a shift in one's occupation. For those fortunate enough to be at the start of their careers, the possibilities are wide open. Longtime vegans with established professions are more often already involved in ethically compatible work. Yet, because veganism is a belief system that necessitates ongoing intentional growth and awareness, changing jobs or training for a new career may be, for some, a natural and integral part of the vegan evolutionary process.

COMPANION ANIMALS

Vegans and animal advocates generally choose to refer to domesticated animals as companions rather than pets because the term *pet* is patronizing and condescending and implies a master-slave or other dominant-subordinate relationship. Vegans are not united in their view of companion animals, making the issue complex. While some believe that dogs, cats, and other domesticated animals should not be in our homes at all, others find that sharing their lives with animals is mutually rewarding, satisfying, and beneficial.

For dogs and cats who live in loving, responsible homes, domestication has its advantages. These animals may be very happy and healthy and live long, wonderful lives. Conversely, millions of dogs and cats are killed every year in pounds and shelters because there are no homes for them, while breeders, puppy mills, and irresponsible owners continue to propagate animals for profit or pleasure. The heartrending truth is that the number of cats and dogs far exceeds the number of loving homes available to them. Unwanted animals are treated as a nuisance and are often abandoned, abused, or killed. Many misguided people desert unwanted animals in rural areas thinking that someone will find them and take them in or that the animals are capable of fending for themselves. Tragically, these animals are faced with starvation, poisoning, freezing, highway death, procurement for research laboratories, and persistent, unrestricted breeding, which only exacerbates the problem.

Animal control agencies and shelters take in several million animals a year, but most cannot house and support all these animals until their natural deaths so healthy animals who are not quickly adopted (in about a week) are killed. In many areas where a practice called pound seizure is permitted, unclaimed animals can be turned over or sold to research laboratories, where their imminent death is preceded by ruthless suffering.

The vast majority of purebred animals sold in pet shops are raised in what are called puppy mills, breeding kennels notorious for their cramped, crude, and filthy conditions and their continuous breeding of unhealthy and hard-to-socialize animals. Animals from puppy mills are bred for quantity, not quality. Continuous in-breeding causes unmonitored genetic defects (such as hip dysplasia), illness and disease (such as parvo and feline leukemia), and personality disorders (such as extreme destructiveness, aggression, antisocial behaviors, and excessive barking). Purchasing a purebred animal perpetuates the endless cycle of breeding for profit. A more reasonable and humane alternative is to seek out a loving companion animal that is already in a shelter and in desperate need of a home. Status breeds and the most expensive animals don't necessarily make the best companions. Often the less glamorous or plainer-looking mixed breeds have the best personalities and temperaments and make the best friends.

Of the unwanted dogs and cats that are abandoned or killed in animal shelters each year, many are purebreds. There is simply no reason for companion animals to be bred. Spaying or neutering is a onetime expense that costs less than raising puppies or kittens and is much lower than the cost that communities must pay for animal control and euthanasia. The vegan population is divided over the ethicalness of subjecting companion animals to surgery (spaying and neutering) based on non-life-threatening conditions. It could be construed that this forced surgery contradicts one of the basic tenets of animal rights—that each living being has a right to her or his own body without imposition. However, as this debate continues, it is critical that vegans weigh all the issues carefully and make sensible decisions based on existing circumstances and realistic consequences.

Another concern facing vegans who adopt dogs and cats is what to feed them. The commercial pet-food industry thrives on the by-products, castaways, and rejects from animal agriculture, using slaughterhouse refuse and diseased or contaminated dregs deemed unsuitable for human consumption. Dogs are carnivorous but are able to eat a wide range of foods. Therefore, some can adapt to a nutritionally well-balanced vegetarian or vegan diet. Commercial vegetarian dog foods and biscuits are readily available, and some mixes can even be prepared at home from blends that incorporate appropriate supplementation of protein, calcium, vitamin D, and crucial amino acids to safeguard the health of your dog. There is much debate, however, over whether or not a vegetarian or vegan diet is appropriate for cats under any circumstances. Whether your companions are dogs or cats, always consult your veterinarian before starting them on a vegan or vegetarian diet.

Cats' physiology is clearly carnivorous, and some veterinarians feel that a cat's health could be endangered or its life jeopardized by a totally vegan regimen. Some vegans compromise by feeding their feline companions a vegetarian diet at home and then allowing them to hunt freely outdoors, stalking, catching, and eating birds, rabbits, mice, chipmunks, squirrels, and other small animals to fulfill their need for meat. However, there are multiple problems with this approach.

Humane agents know that the safest place for domesticated animals is inside the home or, as in the case of dogs, in a fenced yard or on a leash accompanied by their human caregivers. Cats cannot be walked on a leash like a dog, and fences generally do little to contain them. Collars and long leads are very dangerous for cats and can lead to choking or strangulation. Cats are extremely territorial and, when left to roam on their own, typically get into fierce fights with other cats, which can be debilitating, mutilating, or fatal. Uncontrolled interaction with other cats can also lead to unlimited breeding and transmission of lethal viruses and other diseases. Alone and unsupervised, they become easy targets for abuse, poisoning, highway death, impoundment, confiscation, and sale to laboratories. Cities, towns, and even wooded areas are not natural habitats for domesticated cats and dogs; consequently, accidents are rampant. Furthermore, the predation of cats and dogs on unsuspecting birds, small urban mammals, and other native species is cruel and dangerous. The dog or cat can be maimed or injured in the fray, and the consumption of wildlife can spread disease, illness, and rabies. Larger animals that attack smaller ones often mutilate or incapacitate them, then leave them to agonize a slow, lingering death. Animals that wander on their own also pick up fleas, ticks, and other parasites and bring them home to their human families.

According to Zoe Weil, author of *So, You Love Animals* and *Animals in Society,* the ideal world from a vegan perspective might include two different scenarios: one in which companion animals are slowly phased out through a ban on breeding, and another in which humans learn responsible care and establish breeding bans that prevent overpopulation and needless death of these gentle and loving animals.

UNINVITED GUESTS

Much to our chagrin, ants, spiders, mice, bats, squirrels, and other unexpected critters occasionally take up residence in our homes and offices. Although some people might set deadly traps or scatter poisons that cause great suffering, this is not the vegan way. The vegan ethic forbids intentionally killing or harming any sentient being, no matter what species or how tiny. Small intruders, such as rats and mice, are viewed as pests, not pets, and therefore have few defenders; nevertheless, the pain they feel is certainly as real as that of any other animal.

It can be a frustrating challenge to convince these little ones to leave your space, but a good offense is the best defense. To deter mice, rats, and other rodents, maintain clean, sanitary conditions and plug holes or cracks where they might enter. Seal all foods in airtight jars, tins, and other similar containers. The smell of food will lure insects and rodents, and the sharp, strong teeth of mice and rats can easily chew through paper, plastic, and cellophane. Don't leave dirty dishes in the sink or have open pails of garbage or compost in or near the house.

If you have an infestation of rodents, and traps are needed to remove them, use humane box-type release traps (available from mail-order sources, humane societies, and hardware stores). These traps have a door that is triggered shut when the animal enters. The trap can then be taken outdoors, where the animal can be released unharmed. When using these traps, be sure to check them every few hours, because frightened rodents have a high metabolism rate and will quickly become thirsty and hungry.

To prevent an infestation from recurring or to discourage a wide range of insects, rodents, and other critters (such as fleas, ticks, moths, spiders, crickets, bats, and squirrels) from entering your home or office, you can purchase ultrasonic repellers (available through mail-order sources, hardware stores, humane societies, and "green" stores). These electronic devices emit a range of high-frequency sounds that are audible and irritating to specific animals and insects but are beyond the range of human hearing. Most small insects can be gently captured in your hand, taken outdoors, and released.

Read as much as possible to learn about the particular species you are dealing with and take personal safety precautions whenever appropriate. Since the desired results will most likely not happen overnight, any humane removal program calls for patience. It also calls for a gentle touch. Keep in mind that these beings are significantly smaller than we are and often are a lot more intimidated by us than we are by them.

VEGANIC GARDENING

In the not-too-distant past, widespread chemical-dependent farming and unrestrained agricultural genetic manipulation was limited to the fantastic imaginings of science-fiction enthusiasts. Modern science has changed all that. Today, commercially grown fruits and vegetables are commonly tainted with pesticides, herbicides, and other toxic chemicals. Moreover, scientists have inserted animal genes into the genetic code of many fruits and vegetables to create even more attractive produce with greater disease resistance and an abnormally extended shelf life. Because biotech crops are not required by the United States Department of Agriculture or the Food and Drug Administration to be labeled as genetically altered, vegans and vegetarians are unable to know if their produce is totally plant-based or a strange amalgam of plants and animals.

In an effort to maintain agricultural integrity, maximize nutrition and flavor, build soil fertility, and phase out or eliminate chemical-dependent farming practices, there has been a growing trend of U.S. farmers back toward organic farming. It makes sense to cultivate and buy organically grown foods (locally grown, if possible), for several reasons:

1. Organic foods are produced without the use of synthetic pesticides, fertilizers, or growth hormones.
2. Organic farmers promote biological diversity through soil conservation and renewal, crop rotation, and the use of natural fertilizer and pest control.
3. Organic farming helps to maintain the health of our soil, air, and water supplies.
4. Organic farming provides a safer work environment for those who grow our food.
5. Organic farming encourages the use of composting, which, if implemented on a large scale, would significantly reduce the amount of refuse that ends up in our landfills.
6. Organically grown food tastes better.

One of the concerns vegans have with organic farming, however, is the widespread use of dried animal blood, bone meal, manure fertilizers, and other animal-based soil enhancers. Lisa Robinson Bailey describes her surprise when she first learned that animal products are systematically used to grow organic fruits and vegetables:

> My interest in gardening prompted me to take a tour of local organic farms sponsored by the Carolina Farm Stewardship Association. The tour brought home to me the prevalence of using animal products in the production of plant foods. I realized that, even though I was buying organic produce, slaughter-industry by-products like manure from factory farms and bone meal and blood were routinely used to produce my food. It was quite an eye-opener!

Animal products and manure used in composting for application to the soil are inherently dependent on animal husbandry, and utilizing them directly supports the food-animal industry. They are unpleasant to handle, often harbor intestinal, parasitic, and other diseases, may contain antibiotic and other drug residues, and are highly acidic and therefore may require heavier applications of dolomite or lime. Alternatively, soil that is built with plant residues is enriched with natural products produced by earthworms and the abundant minute animal life it directly supports.

The concept of veganic gardening—growing food organically without the use of animal products or by-products—has been in existence for several decades in the United States and parts of Europe, but publications about it are still extremely sparse and scattered. English author Geoffrey L. Rudd coined the term *veganic* in the 1940s. The method was popularized around the same time by Rosa Dalziel O'Brien. She, along with her son, wrote books on veganic gardening, which were published in England.

A variety of gardening techniques used by veganic gardeners include composting with pure vegetable matter; mulching; turning crops under; weeding; soil enhancement and fortification through planned crop rotation; natural insect control through complementary planting; terraced gardens to enhance moisture retention and minimize erosion; and many others. Successful veganic gardening may require a bit of research, creativity, strategizing, and hard work, but your efforts will yield safe, compassionate, and nutritious results.

OF PRINCIPLE AND PRACTICE

The greatest hope for a more peaceful, just, nonviolent, loving world lies with each of us striving to bring alive in every aspect of our individual lives the compassion and understanding that forms the foundation of veganism.

—BRIAN GRAFF

DEGREES OF COMPASSION

Becoming vegan has sensitized me to the feelings of all my fellow beings. I can truthfully say that being a vegan has made me a more compassionate person. If, as the Buddha said, "eating meat extinguishes the seed of compassion," then the converse is true: Being a vegan fosters the growth of the seed of compassion that is within all of us.

—RYNN BERRY

Embracing veganism compels practitioners to confront their attitudes and responsibilities toward all forms of life. Compassion is the emotion that allows us to relate to the feelings of others and inspires us to understand their experiences.

When we confirm that others feel pain, pleasure, and the urge to live, we are moved to acts of altruism and benevolence. There are many different kinds of compassion, however, depending on who the "others" happen to be.

1. *Linear compassion* is what we feel for friends, family, spouse/partner, and children, those with whom we are emotionally close and who are most like us. The bond is reciprocal, allowing empathy to flow back and forth. The output of compassion is directly proportional to the input and is mutually gratifying.

2. *Parallel compassion* applies to people who are similar to us but outside of our immediate realm. They may be individuals or groups we know remotely or have never met but with whom we feel we share a connective bond. For example, parallel compassion can include empathy for people of the same religion, ethnicity, or subcultural group; people who have survived an ordeal together; people who have a similar lifestyle or occupation (such as mothers, homosexuals, students); people who have endured comparable tragedies or challenges (such as illness, a car accident, rape, a disabled child); or neighbors who live in close proximity. Parallel compassion can also extend to those we know little about but with whom we connect on an altruistic plane, such as the children of strangers, homeless people, oppressed groups, victims of crime, or victims of war or other crises (such as famine, floods, tornadoes, etc.). This is a more selfless but removed form of compassion, founded on a detached sense of justice for those with whom we have something in common—our collective humanity. Although this form of compassion is unilateral, it is nevertheless emotionally satisfying to know that others similar to us may benefit from our concern.

3. *Perpendicular compassion* extends to nonhuman animals who are close to us. It requires direct personal interaction. Through this one-on-one association, we discover and acknowledge that, in spite of enormous differences (dissimilar bodies, disparate ways of communicating, etc.), which make it difficult to confirm the other's experiences and perceptions, we can learn to care for each other based on mutual affection and a common link of shared experience found at the point where our lives intersect.

4. *Circular compassion* is what we feel for nonhuman animals with whom we have no direct contact and very little in common. It is similar to parallel compassion in that it contains the element of altruism and there is no direct reciprocation. It, too, stems from a remote sense of justice based on concern for other living beings. However, this type of compassion is one-dimensional. People who practice circular compassion do not extend their compassion to *all* living beings. Their compassion is directed only toward specific groups or species of animals who are designated as important, valuable, endangered, or in need of human assistance or intervention. An example of circular compassion is a fund-raiser picnic sponsored by a no-kill animal shelter where hamburgers, hot dogs, or even a pig are barbecued and served to supporters.

5. *Spherical compassion* is for all living beings, human and nonhuman, near or far, alike or different. It is the recognition that all sentient life is interconnected and that all of our actions, both direct and indirect, impact the welfare and well-being of similar and dissimilar others. Spherical compassion is the essence of veganism.

ETHICAL EFFICACY

Veganism, like compassion, is a matter of the heart, not the head. Few people are convinced to become vegan, and remain so, based strictly on intellectual argument.

Facts and figures change, but ethics based on right and wrong do not. This is not to say that all decisions made by vegans are explicitly predetermined by a rigid ethical code. There are many enigmatic and ambiguous areas, which require deep consideration before an appropriate vegan choice can be made. When confronted with difficult decisions, we must weigh and examine all factors. Matters that present a clear-cut vegan option can be readily resolved. Others, however, may require some level of compromise tempered with the recognition that, because this is not a perfect world, it is sometimes impossible to find a perfect solution. As a result, vegans are occasionally obliged to choose between the lesser of two evils.

There are people who believe that we should all do things in moderation. In terms of compassion, however, what does that mean? Does it suggest that racism is acceptable ten days out of the month as long as you do not engage in it the other days? Does it imply that it's okay to kick the dog on Thursdays and Saturdays if you don't kick him the rest of the week? Does moderation make it acceptable to fire a gun at people as long as it's only occasionally or only people of a certain race, sex, or religion?

Of course not. These examples sound ridiculous because we know that when we believe certain actions to be immoral or unethical, there is no compromise, and moderation seems absurd. Veganism is an ethical practice which, like compassion, cannot be turned off and on for convenience.

Why is it then that the ethical application of veganism frequently does not occur to people who display parallel, perpendicular, and even circular forms of compassion? And why do some who intellectually embrace veganism resist practicing it and continue engaging in activities that exploit certain animals? The answers can be found in the cultural assumption that people should not be forced to sacrifice individual pleasures and familiar patterns. Hence, for these people, spherical compassion becomes acceptable only if it does not impinge on their individual comfort, habits, or cravings. Of course, like most worldviews, this often is not a reasoned conviction but rather an unarticulated, perhaps even unconscious belief.

> The most challenging aspect of being a vegan is confronting every day of your life the fact that you are most definitely in the minority and that no matter how unbelievable it seems, other people may simply not care that the food they eat comes from animals that suffered and felt agonizing pain. This can be very disheartening. One would think that as soon as others' eyes were opened to animal suffering, they would start to make concrete steps toward eliminating animal products from their diet. But oddly enough, otherwise kind, gentle, openhearted people still eat meat and use animal products. I am baffled by it daily.
>
> —Hillary Morris

CONSISTENCY OF CONVICTION

Practice what you preach.

—AMERICAN PROVERB

People who profess to be animal advocates yet eat meat, eggs, or dairy products or wear leather shoes and belts apply contrary rules of ethics. They are practicing circular compassion, also known as selective compassion. Their actions imply that one group of animals—the one they represent—has a greater right to life than another and suggest that sacrificing habit, fashion, beauty, comfort, or taste is a worse evil than taking an animal's life or making an animal suffer. Vegans who encourage congruity are not necessarily extolling a holier-than-thou virtue. Vegan consistency is (or ought to be) nothing less than spherical compassion in action—an abiding intellectual awareness and conscious application of the vegan ethic rather than an exercise in moral or spiritual superiority.

> *Veganism has made me more conscious of behavior patterns that are not consistent with my adherence to philosophic veganism. Being vegan has not made my personality more peaceful, as by some sort of physiological or mystical transformation or holistic purification; however, it has made me intellectually more aware of my feelings and behavior and less able to rationalize and do certain things that I might otherwise overlook.*
>
> —KAREN DAVIS

Undoubtedly, there is complicity in contradictory words and actions, and it undermines the significance and purpose of ethical practice. Every day we make innumerable choices that have a far-reaching impact on others. If we opt to selectively employ our ethics because they are, at times, inconvenient, it invalidates our sincerity. Vegans can consciously *choose* to advance compassion through consistent, unmitigated application of vegan principles in all that they do.

I've been accused of being a do-gooder as though it were a bad thing to be. My reply is that in every situation you can do good, do bad, or do nothing. There are no rules, no laws, no guards looking over your shoulder. You have to let your conscience be your guide.

—Maureen Koplow

People outside of social movements or subcultures often view individual members of a movement or subculture as spokespeople, representatives, or prototypes who embody all the ideal qualities of their cause. Although some people would strongly prefer not to be cast in this role, being placed in this position, even inadvertently, can be a powerful tool for influencing the behavior of others.

Setting and practicing a standard of compassion is not only personally rewarding; it can also bring deep satisfaction from knowing that when others adopt a vegan lifestyle because of your influence, they are enriching their own lives as much as they are helping to eliminate cruelty and suffering.

A sincere and honest effort to maintain vegan consistency is paramount in establishing a credible and honorable vegan presence, regardless of how close an individual actually comes to achieving that goal. Making right choices is not always easy and certainly not always clear-cut. Even when we strongly desire to do good, there is a point where we must accept our limitations or inadequacies and move on. Regardless of one's level of determination or intent, there will be gray areas, times when we unwittingly cross the line, and occasions when we cause harm inadvertently.

SOCIAL BACKLASH

I've been a rebel of sorts all my life, having been taught at an early age that just because it is fashionable to follow the crowd does not mean that happiness or, more important, inner joy will result.

—Roshan Dinshah

It is not easy to be different, and few people choose to be pariahs. Vegans are constantly under enormous pressure to conform from family, friends, colleagues, the media, and blatant as well as unarticulated cultural assumptions. There is comfort in familiarity and complacency, and a vegan approach rattles the status quo. It is always unsettling for people to have their worldview challenged, and a vegan's mere presence can do just that.

Cultural, ethnic, racial, and religious affiliations influence how individuals and groups view veganism. There are those who believe that there are more important problems—racism, homelessness, drugs, violence, poverty, and child abuse, for example—that must be taken care of before we can turn our attention to issues involving animals. Some groups are so immersed in solving their own problems that they believe concerns over seemingly unrelated issues (such as animals or the environment) are baseless, or irrelevant, or have nothing to do with them directly and are therefore unimportant. There are also those who believe that animals are so inferior to humans that the matter shouldn't even warrant our attention. Of course, matters of compassion are not mutually exclusive. It is not a question of helping humans or helping other animals. One can do both.

Oppressed and disempowered people sometimes designate a subordinate role to animals because animals are easy targets for subjugation. Maintaining power over animals reverses the tyrannical roles—the oppressed becomes the oppressor. Hence, by dominating animals, some disenfranchised people can feel that at least on a certain level they are superior to *something*. Regrettably, this attitude can open the door to accepting and even encouraging cruelty, abuse, and killing of animals, which is often a precursor to other forms of violent and heinous behavior.

Because the issues that motivate one to veganism deal with matters of right and wrong and life and death, discussing vegan concerns can make nonvegans feel edgy, ashamed, threatened, or defensive, even when the conversation is not directed at them personally. This can produce tensions in professional, social, and personal relationships, causing vegans to feel guarded and wary of interactions with nonvegans. Protectiveness emanating from both sides creates awkward and uncomfortable communications that have the potential to become hurtful.

Being vegan has made it even more difficult to relate to my family and extended circle of friends, who, for the most part, do not understand my choice to be vegan, or choose not to understand because it would require them to reassess their own choices.

—Jeffrey Brown

Some vegans prefer to avoid the issue of their veganism entirely rather than face a difficult confrontation with a meat eater. A teacher who has been vegan for ten years told me, "Essentially, I have been living a lie on my present job for the past three years. In my classroom, I have had the same teacher's aide for all three years. She does not even know I am a vegetarian, let alone vegan. My ethics caused so many difficulties on previous jobs that I took the easy way out and said nothing. The people with whom I work marvel at my willpower because of all the foods I pass up!"

Over the years, I have heard a variety of responses in reaction to the announcement that someone is vegan or vegetarian. Up until a few years ago, the standard nonvegetarian reply would be "But where do you get your protein?" About five to ten years ago, the rejoinder changed to "But where do you get your calcium?" In the last several years it has shifted to "Well, I only eat a little chicken," or "I only eat a little fish," or "I never eat red meat anymore," or "I'm trying to eat more vegetables." Most vegans and vegetarians I have spoken with feel that the meat eaters who respond this way are seeking a congratulatory response for their "enlightened" eating habits. Nevertheless, from an ethical perspective, the chickens and fish are not grown from seeds and therefore are equally as dead as red meat. Moreover, the fact that someone is eating more vegetables certainly does nothing to help the animals she or he persists in consuming.

The most fascinating aspect of this evolving repartee is that some meat eaters now appear remorseful about continuing to eat meat, often sounding apologetic. This may be a result of feeling guilty, embarrassed, or ashamed that they are eating foods that they believe (or that they think the vegan believes) are unhealthful, or that they know in their hearts are products of pain, suffering, and death. Of course, it could also be that vegans and vegetarians inadvertently bring out feelings of contrition just by their proximity.

RECOILING AND REBOUNDING

Misinformed journalists and so-called culinary experts who evaluate food strictly from a gourmet or health perspective have bastardized the term *vegetarian*. Its 150-year-old definition never included nor was intended to include meat, fish, or fowl of any kind. Yet, today there are "authorities" claiming that it is perfectly acceptable for people who include small amounts of meat in their diet to call themselves semivegetarians. They profess that there are different types of vegetarians: pescovegetarians (those who eat fish), pollovegetarians (those who eat birds), and, if we really want to extend the absurdity, porcovegetarians (those who eat pigs), beefovegetarians (those who eat cattle), and so on. In recent times, the term *vegetarian* has become progressively muddled and hollow.

> Vegans are serious about the ethics surrounding the grand consumption controversy. The word vegetarian holds almost no ethical meaning. Many of us have heard, "I'm a vegetarian but I eat fish." (Those rare ovolacto-ichthyo vegetarians.) The whole concept of being vegetarian has been reduced to a somewhat vague dietary description. Even strict vegetarians, those who eat no animal products at all, will generally wear leather or use other nonfood animal products. A vegan seeks an existence involving the least amount of animal exploitation possible. It is a philosophical ideal that is somewhat more tenable than is possible simply by eating no meat.
>
> —DAVID SMITH

Considering that most meat eaters also include fruits and vegetables in their diets, what makes them any different from these so-called meat-eating vegetarians? Absolutely nothing, of course. Why then would someone want to lay claim to the title of vegetarian if she or he cannot observe its meaning? Perhaps, at long last, the word *vegetarian* has come to signify something desirable, a goal that people strive to attain. If this is the case, it would be more accurate and forthright to express that "I would like to be a vegetarian but have not yet achieved that objective." To distort the meaning of the term *vegetarian* is insensitive to those who created the word and to those who truly practice vegetarianism. As Howard Lyman, former cattle rancher and beef feedlot operator turned vegan, and author of the best-selling book *Mad Cowboy,* tells his audiences, "Don't talk the talk if you can't walk the walk."

Although it is tempting to those who are exceptionally passionate about their beliefs—whether they are of a religious, ethical, philosophical, or social nature—moralizing has never been particularly popular or well-received among the masses. We are all somewhat self-righteous about our own viewpoints, and few among us appreciate being told we may have it all wrong. Recent converts to any belief system or practice are often especially zealous in their enthusiasm and desire to spread the good word. New vegans are no exception. Seasoned vegans, on the other hand, generally come to realize the futility of pontificating and thus seek more constructive ways of conveying the vegan message.

> Preaching the gospel of a vegan lifestyle used to be a mild crusade, but now I seldom draw attention to it. I have found that setting a quiet example is often the best approach; if someone is not ready for change and is not seeking the truth, no amount of logic or appeals to compassion can awaken her or him.
>
> —Kai Wu

Spherical compassion is at the heart of vegan practice and embodies the reverence, caring, and grace extended to all life. Enmeshed in this web of concern, however, is a fusion of both lovable and not-so-lovable individuals. The lovable ones are, of course, a joy to embrace. But reaching out to those who may be abrasive, confrontational, bigoted, violent, abusive, annoying, indifferent, or simply unlike ourselves can sometimes stretch the fibers of this delicate lacework close to the breaking point. Vegan compassion, when exercised to its fullest, can be intricate and challenging, and when uniformly applied, it may prompt even the most enlightened souls to summon their deepest resources for courage, patience, and tolerance.

Lest we overlook an often neglected element of spherical compassion, respect and concern for oneself cannot be stressed fervently enough. In consonance with vegan ideals is learning to understand, accept, honor, nourish, and forgive ourselves no less than we strive to do for others. Too often, compassionate people put themselves and their own needs in the shadows, placing greater importance and merit on helping others. If the self is not included in the practice of vegan principles, then the principles are not being wholly implemented. Taking care of one's needs—physical, mental, social, and emotional—is on a par with all other facets of externally applied activism and must be afforded equal deference and attention, not because it will make you a better activist, or help you live longer in order to further the vegan cause, or any other nebulous rationale, but simply because it is the right thing to do. If the vegan ethic compels one to cherish and revere all life, one must certainly include oneself. *Not* to do so is to violate vegan precepts. *Not* to do so is to do far less than we are capable of doing.

To All My Relations

Peace is the outcome of Love.
Love is the fruit of Compassion.
Compassion is reliant on Caring.
Caring is born of Understanding.
Understanding is contingent on Knowledge.
Knowledge is gained through Perceiving.
Perceiving is based on Observance.
Observance necessitates Awareness.
Awareness requires the ability
to see without eyes,
to hear without ears,
to sense with the heart
and recognize suffering as suffering
regardless of color, culture, language or form.
There is but one sky, one land, one wind, one sea.

We breathe the same air,

sip the same ocean,

share the same portion of time

as we pass through this moment together.

We are children of the Earth,

no less sisters and brothers.

Gather the spurious boundaries that separate our sibling spirits,

for we are family.

Come into my arms, my limbs, my leaves,

and let me stroke your shapeless self.

Let me know your pain.

Let me feel your truth.

Let me embrace our differences,

our sameness,

our uniqueness.

We blend seamlessly, imperceptibly,

distinctions dissolved.

I recognize you now.

Unmasked.

Relieved of our earthly robes,

we are One.

—JOANNE STEPANIAK

ASCENT AND EVOLUTION

Giving up flesh was easy—I became a vegetarian in a single day. But becoming vegan has continued to be a process.

—Maureen Koplow

MODES OF MANIFESTATION

Vegans tend to find the practice of their ethic liberating rather than restricting. Many vegans have told me that once the shackles of an animal-based diet and lifestyle were removed, they discovered that beyond the basic premise of respect for all sentient life was a profusion of additional reasons to be vegan: personal and public health, environmental degradation, world-hunger concerns, social-justice issues, occupational oppression. These grounds may not be enough to motivate an individual toward veganism, but they are viewed by most vegans as adjunct justifications.

The following manifestations of vegan awareness may occur in any order. However, the first three must take place before an individual can fully identify with and fulfill the definition of being vegan. The remaining manifestations may never develop in some people or may evolve over several years or even a lifetime. Occasionally, if someone is exceptionally fortunate, they happen concurrently.

1. Food

Most people begin their vegan journey by changing their diet. In fact, many people who eventually come to veganism start out by first becoming vegetarian. Typically, though not always, milk, cheese, and other dairy products are the last animal-based foods to be excluded from the diet. However, some vegans, especially youths or young adults with passionate enthusiasm, may omit all animal foods at once.

2. Clothing

Often clothing choices are the next logical step in vegan transformation. Some women donate old fur coats to activist groups for anti-fur protests. Other people give their wool coats and sweaters; mohair hats; leather jackets, shoes, gloves, and belts; silk blouses and dresses; and other animal-based clothing and footwear to shelters for the homeless, refuges for battered women and children, and thrift shops. To continue to wear animal fur, hair, and skins, even though the animal may have died long ago, lends credence to the acceptability of using and wearing such items.

Modern society has embraced the concept of clothing as fashion instead of a utilitarian necessity. This has resulted in an annually changing look, to which we must conform to appear in step. As we adopt the new styles, outmoded styles and garments are discarded. Some vegans see this as an obsolete and deleterious custom that encourages an endless cycle of excessive consumption and planned obsolescence. As a result, some vegans choose to shop at thrift stores or wear their current wardrobe for as long as possible, regardless of the latest trends.

Frequently, however, it is not economically feasible or environmentally reasonable to discard all nonvegan clothing at once. For some new vegans, it can take several months or years to cycle out all their animal-based attire.

I must confess that I am still wearing the leather shoes I purchased
before I became vegan, although I haven't bought any leather products

since. Also, I'm still wearing whatever wool sweaters I have. As a grad-
uate student living in a part of the country with long, cold winters, I can-
not afford to replace certain clothing items with cruelty-free products,
and have decided to continue wearing the items I currently own.

—JUDI WEINER

3. Personal Care and Household Items

Switching to vegan personal-care and household products often happens gradually because most people cannot afford to replace a large quantity of goods
at the same time. Also, using up what you already have on hand reduces
wastefulness. Most new vegans replace products one at a time until their
entire house is completely veganized. However, some newcomers may give
away their animal-based products all at once so they can begin their vegan
journey with peace of mind and a clean slate.

4. Human Health

Although health concerns may motivate some people to adopt a vegan-style
diet, for the vast majority of people, health matters are not the reason they
embrace a vegan *lifestyle.* Sooner or later, however, most vegans become aware
of how vegan living can improve their health—both physically and psychologically. This generally does not happen automatically. As with all self-
improvement efforts, it requires a prudent combination of thought, knowledge,
deliberate action, and pragmatic implementation. Some vegans are interested
solely in the altruistic aspects of veganism and don't consider their own health
of particular significance. Others believe that taking care of and extending
compassion to oneself is essential to wholly fulfill vegan principles. As a result,
health matters are often viewed as an ancillary factor in one's choice to be
vegan. Still others neither discount nor extol the health advantages of veganism and accept any benefits they may acquire in stride.

At my age [seventies], a number of my nonvegan friends suffer various
aches and pains. I am fortunate to have none—no heart surgery, no high
blood pressure, etc. I feel happy, energetic, active, and healthy. I have

helped some friends become aware of the benefits of lower-fat vegan eating. They seem to be able to understand about clogged arteries and high blood pressure even when they can't understand about the animals, the rain forest, the soil, or the oceans.

—Shirley Hunting

5. Animal Activism

During the process of becoming vegan, most people also learn about the systemic local, national, and global abuses regularly inflicted upon animals of every ilk. Although working publicly or politically on behalf of animals is not a requirement for being vegan, most vegans eventually become involved in animal advocacy or activism to one degree or another. Furthermore, meat eaters working to alleviate animal use and abuse often become vegan.

6. Environmental Activism

What we eat and how it is produced is inescapably linked to the state of our environment. Many vegans become active environmentalists when they discover that animal agriculture is directly responsible for the bulk of our water usage and pollution, the loss of most of the original topsoil in the United States, the consumption of the majority of all raw materials used in the United States, and the razing of tropical rain forests for cattle grazing, displacing indigenous people and animals and imbalancing ecosystems worldwide.

On occasion, meat-eating environmentalists will become vegan upon realizing that their individual lifestyle choices can have a farther-reaching and longer-lasting impact than most other singular environmental actions. Once vegans acknowledge the connection between diet and the environment, additional "green" lifestyle changes may also be implemented, including recycling; purchasing recycled products and/or buying items with minimal and recyclable packaging; eliminating the use of paper towels and paper plates; composting; gardening; buying only organically (or veganically) grown foods; walking or bicycling instead of driving; shopping for clothes at thrift stores or buying clothes made from recycled materials or organically grown fibers;

installing energy-saving household appliances; supporting environmental organizations; and/or becoming politically active.

7. Social Activism

Because the practice of veganism integrates spherical compassion, it is reasonable that many vegans are also involved with social justice issues concerning oppressed groups of people. Not only do some vegans recognize the remarkable similarities between exploitation of animals and exploitation of humans, research has revealed that abusing, torturing, or killing small animals is often a precursor to other destructive antisocial behavior. Human-rights and animal-rights violations can be powerful motivators for vegans to help break this chain of depravity.

Additionally, vegans are an isolated group, challenging some of our culture's most fundamental assumptions and often being reviled for doing so. Inevitably, many vegans develop an understanding and empathy toward others who are also unjustly castigated.

> I like to think of veganism humbly and holistically. It's about taking personal responsibility in a world so full of needless suffering. It's challenging oneself to open one's eyes and question society's assumptions and habits. It's about critical thinking and compassion and how one would like to see the world evolve.
>
> —Michael Greger

8. Peace Activism

Peace does not always connote the opposite of war, nor does it necessarily signify a state of calm. In some instances, peace may mean the absence of violence and/or a method of settling disputes without inflicting pain. Conflict is inevitable, but we do have a voice in how we resolve it. Because violence on any level causes suffering, people who have embraced spherical compassion have an express interest in establishing peace at all levels.

In addition to working to end the war on animals, vegans may be inspired to work for peace in a variety of ways. Some vegans receive training in alternative dispute resolution or mediation. Their skills can then be used to relieve conflicts locally, nationally, and internationally, including animal- and human-rights abuses, environmental disputes, ethnic conflicts, restorative justice, collaboration and community building, violence prevention, and to facilitate communication between culturally and ideologically diverse groups.

Often vegans also explore the inward realms of peace, recognizing that peaceful acts emanate more freely and profusely from people who are foremost at peace in their hearts. Anger, hatred, jealousy, rage, resentment, and malice are cut from the same cloth; those who wear any of these are cloaked in strife. Therefore, learning how to manage, release, and avoid internal turmoil can be a worthwhile tool for gaining inner peace, as well as for generating external tranquillity, which can radiate far beyond our physical presence and linger long after we depart.

> *Veganism understands that gentleness cannot be a product of violence, harmony cannot be a product of strife, and peace cannot be a product of contention and conflict.*
>
> —Stanley Sapon

9. Enhanced Spirituality

Although vegans come from a variety of religious backgrounds, many find their spiritual beliefs strengthened or intensified by their vegan ethic. Because veganism is so all-encompassing, it is not surprising that its principles form the core value system for a large number of practitioners. Some people refer to veganism as their "religion" because the tenets of vegan practice and belief create a compelling moral code on a par with any religious doctrine or theology.

> *The teachings of traditional religions only make sense to me up to a point. Veganism offers a clarity that I believe is in harmony with the spirit of all religious and spiritual beliefs. But it's much more than a cause for hope; it offers serious and practical answers to many perplexing problems facing individuals and all humanity.*
>
> —Brian Graff

10. Evolving Worldview

Among the most exciting vegan manifestations is the realization that humans are not the center of the universe—that *all* living beings have a rightful place, and we are just one among many. Looking at the world in this new light presents a significantly more intimate perspective of our relationship with the Earth and its other inhabitants, one that can be very exhilarating as well as humbling. This new outlook can conceivably be the impetus for initiating all the above manifestations. It can also be the intuitive outcome of living a vegan life.

> *Veganism is a choice that positively impacts so many aspects of our world—not only the animals, the environment, and physical human health but also the whole spiritual and ethical state of our society. A single person's decision to change and practice a truly compassionate and nonviolent lifestyle touches so many other lives and sets such a wonderful example for building a gentler, more peaceful and ethical world— a world with less suffering, oppression, violence, and pain.*
>
> —SHARI KALINA

LEVELS OF CONSCIOUSNESS

Making the decision to become vegan can feel overwhelming at first. Suddenly, so many seemingly unrelated aspects of life are under scrutiny. Although some people leap into a vegan lifestyle overnight, many who come to veganism do so through a series of steps that may take weeks, months, or even years.

> *I am still becoming vegan as I learn more and more each day. I thirst for information and knowledge. As I become more aware of the results of my actions and make changes accordingly, the more vegan I become.*
>
> *To me, being vegan is not a static state. It is a way of living and a way of looking at life and the world. It is not something that stops or is achieved at a particular point in time.*
>
> —KEVIN PICKARD

For most people, veganism is not an end unto itself; it is an ongoing, active process—a vibrant stream of awareness continually flowing toward greater clarity and refinement. Even once someone attains the outward manifestations of veganism, there are often many more internal evolutions yet to take place. None of us has so reached perfection that we have achieved the vegan ideal. Yet, that is exactly what makes veganism so exciting—there is always more to learn, more to give, more to strive for.

15

EMBRACING THE CHOICE

Allow yourself to think, let yourself understand, free yourself to feel. As much as the heart shapes the deed, the deed can also shape the heart.

—Saurabh Dalal

VEGAN AWAKENING

The purpose of veganism is to create a more just and compassionate society by transforming the fundamental tenets of our culture. Embracing veganism is an extremely personal, sometimes complex choice, originating from one's core values—emanating *from the inside out*. This decision can dramatically alter one's life forever.

The transition to veganism is profound, often producing deep emotional changes. Although choosing veganism is a source of great joy, it can also create friction among family and friends. Cultural pressures, the demand for conformity, and the personal desire for acceptance can challenge a vegan's confidence and self-esteem.

Most vegans go through several stages of psychological adjustment as they adapt to this new way of life. This transformative period can place individuals in a very vulnerable position, caught between the conflicting values of two opposing belief systems. Even long-term vegans occasionally encounter disturbing shifts of emotion. There are several inward processes many vegans experience—often to varying degrees and in varying sequence—as they explore and settle into the compassionate way of life.

TRIALS AND TRIUMPHS

New vegans are typically very impassioned about their beliefs; however, they may be guarded and sensitive about them as well. Although criticism is somewhat easier to withstand when excitement is fresh and strong, all vegans are susceptible to being hurt by reproach from friends and family and would prefer that their veganism be positively affirmed by the people with whom they are closest. Because the vegan ethic guides adherents to a deeper awareness of their internal values, vegans are often inspired to convey their innermost feelings. When received with acceptance, such deep communication can create more meaningful and intimate relationships; when met with intolerance or rejection, the outcome can be disheartening, discouraging, and sometimes emotionally devastating.

Some nonvegans hold preconceived notions about veganism, imposing presuppositions (about one's motivation, appearance, health, finances, interests, intellect, education, career, race, religion, political views, spiritual outlook, sexual orientation, family background, personal history, etc.) that may be unfounded and unfair. Whether stemming from ignorance, intolerance, misinformation, or defensiveness, the results can be humiliating or oppressive. Every vegan is a unique individual endowed with special talents, tastes, quirks, problems, and potential. Baseless typecasting can be insulting at best and cataclysmic at worst. Recognizing the distinctive qualities of vegans, and acknowledging the vegan ethic as the sole coalescing force behind such a diverse group of people, will help eradicate pointless, unproductive, and often hurtful stereotypes.

Many people have preconceived notions about what it means to be a vegetarian—that vegetarians subsist on lettuce and carrot sticks and are undernourished and emaciated—and the concept of veganism doesn't even exist for them. I have always had difficulty with my weight and did experience a significant weight loss when I first became a vegan. But becoming vegan did not resolve my food issues, like eating in response to emotion rather than hunger. I have had nonvegetarians look me up and down in disbelief when I told them I was a vegetarian.

It has been very difficult coming to terms with society's notion of fat and thin and the ideal female body. I know some animal-rights groups promote vegetarianism in their literature as a panacea for weight problems, which I think is a betrayal of activists whose bodies do not reflect this notion. I actually reached my highest body weight ever as a vegan, and I feel it is extremely important that, as vegans, we don't try to capitalize on society's obsession with thinness and dole out the same bill of goods the media does.

—LISA ROBINSON BAILEY

Being vegan is not what others imagine it to be. So many people think I eat this way because I want to be healthy. My health is important to me, but the fate of the animals and the Earth comes before any sense of my personal well-being. It is important for me to make that distinction at whatever level I can.

—IRENE CRUIKSHANK

WEATHERING THE TIDE

Vegans in unsupportive situations can face a monumental struggle to remain true to their beliefs. Those who are surrounded with empathy, understanding, reassurance, and respect are best equipped to make a rapid and successful emotional adjustment.

Even if someone is the only vegan in town, it is possible to abide by his or her convictions. The trick may be to find or develop a network of support outside one's immediate vicinity. Some national organizations list in their publications contact people in cities and towns across the country. These volunteers can be excellent sources of information about local vegan organizations, activities, and restaurants. National activist groups and publications can provide a wealth of helpful information, as well as a calendar of events. Attending conferences and conventions builds a sense of community, inspiration, and solidarity and helps develop friendships far and wide.

New vegans are typically surprised and amazed to discover the expanse of material that is available through local and national groups and organizations, books, publications, activist seminars, protests, conferences, festivals, and Websites. Initial contacts are often stepping stones to even further alliances. Frequently, what one finds is an unexpected plethora of information so extensive it can be somewhat overwhelming.

Having just one other vegan friend or contact may be enough to help someone weather rough periods of feeling alienated or alone. Realizing that vegans are part of a larger community that spans the nation as well as the globe can bring joy, comfort, and relief. The secret to overcoming a sense of estrangement is to take the initiative and reach out. There are many welcoming arms waiting to embrace vegans in need of reassurance, validation, love, and support.

THE VEGAN BLUES

In any normal, healthy life we can expect a few dives to the bottom of the emotional barrel. Short periods of sadness may be unavoidable, but at times they help us appreciate the peak joys of life even more. Despair can become a dysfunction, however, when it is chronic or uncontrollable.

Because vegans so acutely see and feel the suffering in the world and are at odds with many widely accepted social customs, some will invariably experience occasional bouts of the blues. If these brief periods are allowed to run their course, they can be valuable learning experiences, which can propel an individual to greater action and service. Vegans who experience anger, pain, or frustration for extended periods of time may become depressed and exhausted from maintaining such intense emotions. Feelings of loneliness, isolation, or rejection can compound matters, leading to despondency in an otherwise emotionally healthy person.

Although seeking professional help may be appropriate and advisable in some situations, be aware that many social activists experience intermittent lows, and the temporary blues are not unusual or necessarily cause for alarm. It is important for friends and family to encourage their vegan loved ones to develop or become part of a supportive network of like-minded people. Sharing stories helps nonconformists realize they are not alone. Friends and family can also lend support to a vegan loved one by providing a safe, non-judgmental environment in which he or she can vent freely, feel heard, and be understood.

Other ways to demonstrate support include cooking and sharing a vegan meal, attending an activist meeting together, or shopping for vegan food or clothing. Vegans who feel depressed need the active support of their loved ones demonstrated through tangible expressions of concern and understanding that affirm their vegan beliefs.

TIES THAT BIND OR BOND

Holidays and celebrations such as birthdays, weddings, anniversaries, and reunions are opportunities to reconnect with family and friends and feel a part of the broader culture. However, most gatherings center around customs and practices that are very upsetting to vegans. Meat is typically the center of the holiday table and the focal point of picnics and barbecues. Gift exchanges of inappropriate items can be awkward, troublesome, and unwelcome. Although most happy occasions are intended to convey a spirit of fellowship and conviviality, they can be extremely uncomfortable and unpleasant experiences for vegans. Consequently, it is not surprising that many vegans feel torn over their allegiances and may distance themselves from family and community celebrations, opting instead to participate in alternative festivities or start their own traditions with others who share their perspectives and ideals.

> The most difficult challenge for me in being vegan is the separation
> and distance I often feel from others who aren't vegan. It is no longer
> comfortable for me to sit down at a table where animal products are
> served. I feel that I know too much, and it is so painful to be aware of

the profound suffering and misery that is represented on the table. This is especially true at celebrations such as Thanksgiving or Passover when the holiday is about freedom and gratitude. Oppressing and harming others while we speak words of thanksgiving feels hypocritical and wrong to me. Yet, feeling disconnected and separated from friends and family doesn't feel good either.

—Zoe Weil

LOVING ONESELF, LOVING OTHERS

Because veganism challenges adherents to live and let live, it can be a powerful tool for personal growth. The vegan ethic requires practitioners to consider the effect of every thought, word, and action on others and on the Earth. Some vegans believe that a lifestyle that habitually or unconsciously employs cruelty through the use of animal-based foods and products is ultimately dehumanizing and incapable of producing a psychologically sound human being. The theory goes that people who engage in cruelty in one area of their lives are more likely and willing to accept cruelty in other areas as well. Even our language is replete with unwitting expressions revealing our culture's rampant but subliminal disdain of animals.

It has been very difficult overcoming the years and years of indoctrination and cultural socialization which told me that eating the flesh of animals was a good thing and that detachment from the emotional lives of animals and nature in general is desirable. I still struggle to catch myself repeating some of the common antianimal clichés, like "I ate like a pig," or "She is as dumb as a cow," or "Kill two birds with one stone."

—Brian Klocke

At its core, veganism is a philosophy that champions love and peace. Hence, many vegans use their ethic to guide them in reflecting these qualities. New, young, or highly passionate vegans often quickly discover that expressing their viewpoints in an angry or contentious manner only creates hostility.

Conversely, when opinions are explained respectfully and lovingly, others are more likely to listen.

> *I am vegan for reasons of wanting to be nonviolent. It is difficult for me to see people using veganism in militant and aggressive ways toward those who are not vegan. Harmlessness extends to human animals as well.*
>
> —IRENE CRUIKSHANK

Veganism can be one of the most effective and emphatic affirmations of an individual's commitment to self-love—a powerful expression of a deep desire to embrace the life that exists inside ourselves. Self-love can be viewed as a fundamental and natural corollary of the vegan ethic of compassion for all life. Some vegans find a remarkable reciprocity between loving themselves and loving others.

> *The most rewarding aspect of being vegan is that the practice of nonviolence and compassion also includes extending this to myself and increases my ability for self-love and self-acceptance. By doing this, I am able to share more love, compassion, and acceptance with others, no matter what their lifestyle is or the choices they make.*
>
> —SALLY CLINTON

Veganism can also be very self-affirming and empowering. It provides a means of productive expression for the outrage activists feel about the injustices in the world, along with a concrete, constructive mode for creating positive change. Furthermore, veganism offers valuable guidance to practitioners in helping them discover their role and purpose in life.

> *Being vegan has given me a receptacle into which I can put my views of the world. I have a place to put my moral outrage against human cruelty to all species. I have a place to put my fears about the environmental future of this planet. I have a way of looking at the world and saying, This is my place in it.*
>
> —JENNIE COLLURA

Anyone who has been in a relationship with someone who holds fundamentally different values knows how extraordinarily draining, painful, and difficult it can be. Such relationships are no less challenging between vegans and nonvegans, and because veganism affects the very basic, compulsory, and inescapable aspects of daily living—food, clothing, and occupation—it can be even harder. Having a partner who shares your outlook on life, your spiritual perspectives, and your dietary preferences can be incredibly exciting, gratifying, and affirming.

> When I first decided to become a vegan, my then-husband (we have since divorced) was not ready to do the same. That was okay with me. I did not expect anyone else to follow my belief system, but I did not want to be held back from following it myself. I disposed of my leather shoes, bags, belts, etc. My husband became upset, which confused me; I found it difficult to live with his being upset. I wanted him to know that it was okay with me for him to believe differently. I just wanted him to let me follow my beliefs without protest.
>
> —Lorene Cox

> Meeting my wife at a vegetarian conference and getting married one year later was very profound. I'd had a number of relationships that didn't work out because of ethical differences, and having a partner who is also vitally committed to vegan living is the most fulfilling experience of my life.
>
> —David Melina

FELLOWSHIP, FRIENDSHIP, AND THE VEGAN TRIBE

Because veganism is such an enormous step outside traditional cultural norms, it can create rifts and misunderstandings between vegans and their nonvegan friends. Although differing viewpoints could potentially bring new depth to old friendships, frequently the gulf becomes too large or onerous to overcome.

Many people find change hard to accept, especially when it occurs in their friends. New perspectives can be threatening and may force others to question the validity of their own convictions. The more comfortable people are with their belief systems and their values, the greater likelihood they will be able to support radical changes in their friends. However, maintaining friendships when lifestyles have grown so drastically apart can be difficult.

Being vegan has changed my circle of friends, my profession, my hobbies, my religious outlook. . . . For example, I am no longer close to many people who were my friends for years. I have simply lost interest in spending time with them. It's too hard for me. Thus, all my close friends now are at least vegetarian, if not vegan.

—MARIANNE ROBERTS

There is joy and camaraderie in sharing common values; consequently, vegans seek each other out, often creating extensive support networks across thousands of miles. By attending vegan/vegetarian events and animal-rights conferences and communicating by phone, mail, and over the Internet, vegans have found a strong sense of community that links them together regardless of distance. It is this remarkable bond that helps so many vegans maintain their commitment and dedication against incredible odds from an apathetic society.

There is a sense of community and connection I feel with other vegans. I have met the most wonderful people ever, people I probably would not have otherwise met! My reasons for becoming vegan have been enhanced and validated many times over since being around other people who share the same beliefs about living a compassionate life.

—ALAN EPSTEIN

VEGAN VALUES, VEGAN VISION: CREATING A COMPASSIONATE WORLD

Even if you never have any children of your own, you may adopt, provide foster care, or volunteer as a big brother or big sister. If you never become a parent, you still inherit a duty to nurture that which sustains our lives. We also need to parent other life around us—plants and animals, as well as water and wilderness.

—Marcia Pearson

Although the causes of increasing violence, poverty, homelessness (of people as well as nonhuman animals with dwindling habitat), environmental devastation, and pollution are complex, many researchers concede that a number of social problems and ecological imbalances are rooted in excessive human overpopulation. Our reckless and insatiable compulsion to reproduce without constraint has forced industrialized societies to develop or demolish significant portions of the natural world. This has displaced and destroyed indigenous life forms and crowded the remainder to make room for our ever-burgeoning and ever-needy populace. The Earth's ecology was not designed to support such a deluge of humans, and few life-forms, including humans, are capable of withstanding the explosion of a single species. Many vegans decide to help mitigate this crisis by electing not to have children, limiting the size of their families, or choosing to adopt.

Like most people, vegans find a variety of ways to nurture youngsters, whether their own or the children of relatives, friends, or neighbors. Foster parenting and volunteer programs also present endless opportunities to be involved in the lives of young people.

Hope for the future lies in the hands of our children. If they are instilled with the vegan vision of a kinder world where all life is afforded equal consideration and respect, then peace, ecological balance, justice, and harmony stand a reasonable chance. It is not difficult to raise vegan children in today's world—certainly no more of a hardship than being a person of color or belonging to a minority ethnic or religious group. Just as we would not ask someone to dismiss her or his cultural heritage or spiritual beliefs, the same considerations can and should be extended to vegans.

However, maintaining a vegan lifestyle may be particularly challenging for children, adolescents, and even young adults who face tremendous peer pressure to conform. Marcia Pearson is the mother of two adolescent girls who have been vegan "since conception." She is intimately aware of the delights and tribulations of raising vegan children in a nonvegan world. Based on her experiences, Marcia offers this sage advice:

We need to let our children know that there is nothing wrong with being different and that there are lots of people who live as they do but perhaps not in their neighborhood or church or school. We need to remind them that they are fortunate to know about being vegan and teach them about all of the reasons.

Since fitting in is important to children, I recommend linking up with a local vegetarian group so that vegan children can meet other vegan children. If that is not possible, then parents could provide materials that tell stories about being a vegan kid and perhaps set up a pen pal. When you are a fish swimming upstream, and especially a young one, it is nice to know that you are not alone.

For school-age children, planning ahead so that appealing snacks and lunches are readily available can ease some of the stigma of being unique. It may also be necessary for parents to prepare a snack or meal before and possibly after their child goes to a party or special event. If it's feasible to call ahead to the hosts before a child attends a gathering, they may be able to provide a few vegan foods as part of the standard fare so everyone can partake and no one needs to feel peculiar or left out. In addition, a child may feel that her or his clothing or shoes aren't fashionable. Therefore, it is essential for garnering self-esteem that parents and children jointly seek out current styles made from comfortable vegan fabrics and materials.

Perhaps what is most critical in helping vegan children adjust to living in a nonvegan world is for parents to explain to their children *why* they are vegan. Most children have instinctive compassion and a natural affinity for animals, nature, wildlife, and the outdoors. When they understand the roots of harmlessness in their diet and lifestyle, being different can become a source of pride. Also, when teachers, extended family members, the parents of friends, and other adults involved in a child's life are well informed about what veganism means and entails, it will be easier for them to help the child feel comfortable away from home.

It is extremely important to explain to the nonvegan adults involved in a child's life specifically what is and is not suitable to avoid embarrassment or awkwardness when exchanging gifts of food, clothing, and personal items or extending invitations. Teachers, caregivers, and other adults should take precautions to ensure that children are not placed in the uncomfortable position of having to explain their lifestyle, being put on a pedestal, or having unnecessary attention drawn to them simply because they are vegan.

Parents need support also. Although not impossible, it is certainly difficult to lead a vegan life in a vacuum, and raising a vegan child can multiply that challenge significantly. Even if there are no other vegans in one's immediate circle, it is essential to develop a supportive network of either vegetarians who are sympathetic to vegan beliefs or other vegans to communicate with by mail, phone, fax, or E-mail. Surrounding oneself with books and literature can reinforce ethics and reignite motivation. Connecting with a local grassroots animal-rights group, if available, and/or joining a national vegan organization that includes a periodic magazine is another way to feel in touch with like-minded people. Receiving a publication that provides relevant information, mail-order services for books and vegan items, suggestions for meals and snacks, and articles to help strengthen and vitalize vegan convictions will stave off feelings of isolation.

When children understand why their parents have chosen to raise them as vegans, and when they are given a choice in the matter at an appropriate age, vegan children are more likely to grow into healthy, well-adjusted vegan adults. Of course, not all parents are comfortable with allowing young children to make such a significant, profound, and far-reaching decision. Many would prefer waiting until their daughters or sons are older, more mature, and capable of understanding all the ramifications of their choice. Nevertheless, as difficult as it might seem, it may become necessary for parents to stand back from their own emotional and ethical viewpoints in order for their offspring to establish their own values—independent of what the parents think and believe. When ideals are foisted on youngsters, they are more prone to rebel against them and do the complete opposite of what a parent desires. However, when children actively participate in the decision to become vegan, they are more likely to feel it is a choice they can embrace, own, and practice—quite possibly for a lifetime.

REORIENTING THE COMPASS

I love being vegan. I love the word. I love all the decisions I've made, even when they are sometimes less than simple. All the moral and ethical judgments that go along with that decision bolster everything else. It is my religion, my road map, my reason for being. Once you take out an ethical yardstick in one area of your life, for me it's difficult to ignore it everywhere else.

—JENNIE COLLURA

REFLECTING ON MEANING

Although the vegan community is diverse and difficult to classify by standard delineations of age, occupation, religion, race, income, etc., it is fascinating to note that when I asked various people who practice veganism to define the term *vegan,* nearly everybody incorporated her or his own unique twist, gently tugging at the parameters established by both the British Vegan Society and the American Vegan Society. There was an invisible thread connecting the underlying thoughts of everyone I spoke with. No one contradicted the original definitions; they simply interpreted the application of the definitions to their lives in significantly broader ways.

Many people I spoke with feel that compassion toward human as well as nonhuman animals is an essential component of being vegan. Others commented on vegans' commitment and responsibility to the Earth and the environment. Most believe that the term *vegan* encompasses more than just one's outward behavior; some refer to it as a philosophy, a lifestyle, a process, a consciousness, an ethic, a perspective, or a truth. Following are some representative responses.

> *For me, the term* vegan *signifies a way of living that liberates humans and animals from centuries of mutual enslavement. Veganism is more than a dietary regime; it is a way of life that promises a richer and nobler existence for all creatures small and great.*
>
> —Rynn Berry

> *Vegan—respectful and positive with a sincere desire toward the uncompromisingly ethical.*
>
> —Saurabh Dalal

> *Being vegan means one is not contributing to animal exploitation and animal slavery. It means living as lightly on the Earth as possible, a higher consciousness, a greater sensitivity to all life forms, human and animal.*
>
> —Shelton Walden

> *Being vegan is a life- and spirit-altering, all-encompassing ethic based on the recognition of and respect for all sentient life.*
>
> —Michael Stepaniak

> *To me, veganism is a lifestyle choice based on the principle of ahimsa, or nonviolence. It is more than a diet. It is something that affects every aspect of my life, from the food I eat, the products I buy, and the clothes I wear, to my thoughts, actions, and relationships with other people, animals, and the planet. Being vegan also means accepting and being tolerant of others' choices while still being true to what I believe and feel is right.*
>
> —Sally Clinton

A CONCEPT AND A DEFINITION REVISITED

The founders of the vegan movement did an incredible job pioneering the framework and providing the guidance for what has become a thriving international campaign for justice and compassion. The word *vegan* has come to be known and understood worldwide. Yet there is some discrepancy between the formal definition of *vegan* and the way it is construed by many of today's practitioners.

With concern for this disparity, I consulted with Stanley Sapon, Ph.D., retired professor of psychology and psycholinguistics, a seventeen-year vegan, and an internationally renowned authority on the psychology of language. I asked him if he thought it would be sacrilegious to revisit the vegan societies' definitions, not with the intent of replacing them but to build upon their strong foundation. Sapon responded:

> Definitions reflect the insights and understanding of the original thinkers. When a group's vision is set by a definition, we need to take care that the perspectives of the era in which the definition was formulated have not become carved in stone, taking on a kind of scriptural immutability. Realities change, and our guidelines need to be responsive and accessible to those changes.

Some vegans told me they are uncomfortable with the idea of trying to define the word *vegan* in the first place because the definition could be restrictive, exclusionary, or even elitist.

In response, Sapon elaborated on the purpose of definitions in general and what they can and cannot accomplish:

> Definitions can be guiding, inspiring, and liberating in some settings, and in others, they can be taken as limiting, restrictive, and coercive. They can tell what you are free to do, or what is forbidden.
>
> We look in the dictionary to help us define words. That same dictionary shows us that groups of people can also be defined—that is, characterized and distinguished from other groups. The word *definition* comes from the Latin *definire,* which means to establish boundaries, to draw lines around specific

territories. A definition based on beliefs or values can be said to mark the boundaries—to draw a kind of map of the ethical territory we aspire to inhabit.

When definitions serve to identify and describe the body of values around which people gather, they also serve to present that body of values as a model and an ideal. In this sense, a clear description of an ethic, a set of ideal moral principles, or a goal can serve as a guidepost, a way of setting one's behavioral compass.

How we define ourselves can certainly affect the way we interact among ourselves. This same issue of definition affects how others will treat us, presetting their expectations concerning us and the kinds of predictions they make about our behavior.

In light of this analysis, I asked Sapon if he thought augmenting the definition of *vegan* might be relevant and/or beneficial to the modern movement. Sapon replied:

> It is vital to acknowledge that it is the sense of *community* that confirms feelings of comradeship, mutual support, and celebration of a shared core of values and ideals. It cannot be some higher authority that determines what behavior will be considered within or outside the boundaries of the vegan ideal; it must be a strong internal consensus of moral judgment.
>
> We need to lay to rest the specter of the holier-than-thou image of vegans that has intimidated many people. It is a simple matter of fact—not comparative virtue—that some people resonate more keenly than others to certain issues. We vegans expect that our characterization of veganism will raise people's consciousness. From that new vantage point, new perceptions are possible, new insights may be generated, and still higher levels of consciousness may be reached.
>
> When our definitions make our values, goals, and ideals more explicit, we add a dynamic spirit to the evolution of ideas, and strength to the vegan movement.

Based on our discussion, I asked Sapon if he would be willing to devise an interpretation that would encompass and reflect the perspective of the vast majority of vegans with whom I spoke—an explanation that would acknowledge the allied *motivation* behind vegan behavior and incorporate with equal weight the concerns for human and nonhuman justice and ecological preservation. I also inquired if it would be possible to create a definition that embodied the spirit of the original definition but was less proscriptive. This is not to imply that the behavior of vegans should be more permissive or indulgent. However, many vegans find it peculiar and perturbing to be defined by what they *don't* do rather than by what they *do* and what they *believe*. Sapon obliged, and the following is the outcome of his efforts based on my suggestions and our joint communications.

EXPANDING THE SPHERE

The following definition, conceived by Stanley Sapon, Ph.D., stems from many people's yearning to have the meaning of veganism put into positive terminology that is prescriptive instead of prohibitive. It was designed to be used, along with its associated code of ethics, as an adjunct to the definitions put forth by The Vegan Society and the American Vegan Society. This interpretation and its predecessors are complementary, not divisive. When used separately or in conjunction with each other, they address and resolve most questions and concerns regarding vegan living.

> Veganism is an ethic that is committed to reverence and respect for all life and the planet that sustains it. Veganism brings with it the joy of living with peace of spirit, and the comfort of knowing that one's thoughts, feelings, words, and actions have a strongly benevolent effect on the world.

A CODE OF VEGAN ETHICS

People who live by vegan principles employ the following code of ethics:

- Vegans are sensitive to issues of suffering; therefore, vegans shun actions that inflict pain, whether intentionally or thoughtlessly, on sensate, animate life, animal or human.
- Vegans value the uniqueness of all life forms; therefore, vegans seek to

avoid wanton destruction of plant life and the exploitation of the physical environment in ways that endanger local or global ecosystems.

- Vegans abjure violence; therefore, vegans seek to deal with physical and social challenges in ways that are thoughtful, gentle, compassionate, considerate, and just.
- Vegans expand the principle of harmlessness; therefore, vegans strive for active beneficence by performing acts of kindness or charity.

Among the ways that vegans manifest their commitment to this code of ethics:

- Vegans choose foods that are exclusively plant-based.
- Vegans explicitly withhold economic and moral support from enterprises that exploit or abuse animals or humans.
- Vegans take care to choose those materials and products that neither destroy nor distort the lives of sensate creatures.
- Vegans actively reject the use of living creatures as instruments or materials for teaching, scientific inquiry, entertainment, or other utilitarian purposes.

CHALLENGES, GIFTS, AND OFFERINGS

I cannot think of a single way that being vegan has not changed my life. From my professional career, to my personal relationships, to my view of the physical universe and my role in it, becoming vegan has created a validity, a focus, a compass guide, and a gold standard for my entire life's journey.

—Michael Klaper

I asked a number of vegans about the concerns and difficulties presented by a vegan lifestyle and the rewards and blessings they have received. It could easily be argued that one should not be rewarded or seek rewards simply for *not* doing acts that are considered unethical, immoral, or just plain wrong. However, it could also be asserted that because most North Americans accept as normal those actions that vegans deem immoral, vegans hold an exceptionally unique perspective of the culture and its inequities and iniquities. Vegans are keenly aware of the many practices they abhor and why. Few moral decisions are so profound, since vegans are continually surrounded by those same violent behaviors they renounce and repudiate. Being inescapably exposed to nonvegan values in essence becomes a constant reminder of the serenity and grace of vegan living.

I also extended an invitation to this group to submit any comments they wished to share with nonvegans and/or new vegans. The following sample of their thoughts and feelings demonstrates the range of their diversity, as well as the parallel thinking that is shared by vegans the world over.

THE CHALLENGES OF BEING VEGAN IN A NONVEGAN WORLD

The most difficult challenge of being vegan is living in a society that is so un-vegan and materialistic. The lives of animals (including humans) are not considered sacred and have become increasingly commodified.

—GENE BAUSTON

Apart from eating out less, being vegan isn't really a challenge. Sometimes getting animal-free clothing is a little tough—but it's not much harder than shopping for exactly what you want.

—DAVID SMITH

Those of us who are vegan choose to be vegan—we can't whine about how difficult it is. We accept a few challenges because it's worth it. If it were such a big boulder on our backs, then we wouldn't carry it.

—MARCIA PEARSON

Cheese! It is definitely an emotional attachment!

—RAE SIKORA

Although food shopping has become increasingly easier in the last twenty years, lack of restaurants that serve vegan food is still a challenge. Interpersonal relationships are challenging with people who are comfortable eating a meat-based diet. I became vegan when I was 57 years old and I am now in my seventies. It is difficult for me to understand people who adamantly state that it's too late for them to make an effort to change.

—RHODA SAPON

REFLECTIONS ON THE REWARDS OF BEING VEGAN

It is rewarding to live with integrity. When I do not live in accordance with my deepest values, I feel a sense of dis-ease and disconnection. The more thoroughly I live my life with integrity and intention, the better I feel.

—ZOE WEIL

I don't think of being vegan in terms of rewards. It's just my way of being in the world. No doubt at the end of the day we can think we've done some good if we've made it through the day as a vegan. Or at least that we've avoided doing some harm. But the contributions our small choices make to the good of the world are mighty small. If there is a reward, it lies in knowing that you've made it through another day doing your best to live the kind of life you think is worth living.

—TOM REGAN

It is hard to talk of the most rewarding aspect of being vegan. In an ocean of good feelings and contentment, it is hard to find the most rewarding drop of water.

—STANLEY SAPON

I find it very rewarding to look at an animal face-to-face and know that peaceful bond between us is real and will not be broken. I am at peace with myself, which makes it more natural to be at peace with others.

—AMY COTTRILL

It is rewarding to realize that life is a miracle and value the excitement of being alive in a way that is free of destruction and violence. Veganism is a way to connect with all that is and be released from the illusion of what we're told we should be.

—MAE LEE SUN

For me, every aspect of being vegan is rewarding. It is almost impossible to narrow the rewards of being vegan down to one element. I have been rewarded with many wonderful vegan friends. I have gained increased vitality for life, not only emotionally and physically but also intellectually and spiritually. I have gained peace of mind from knowing that I have taken and continue to take, every day, new steps toward causing less death and destruction in the world. I have been rewarded with an ever-increasing and creative repertoire of food. And of course my increased understanding and compassion for all of existence has been a great reward as well.

—BRIAN KLOCKE

Being vegan has changed my life immensely—in learning about the way of the world, thinking new and sometimes radically different thoughts, meeting incredible and caring people, and being involved in a movement for social change that simply has to be if the world is to move forward successfully and harmoniously.

—SAURABH DALAL

THOUGHTS FOR NONVEGANS AND NEW VEGANS

Think about your actions. Ponder the interconnectedness of your existence, the Earth, and the other animals who live here. Realize that you are an animal and that the animals you eat, the animals you watch in circuses, the animals you wear, the animals who suffered to produce your cosmetics, all feel pain, love, sadness, and fear, just like you. Recognize that you can eliminate a small part of the suffering by becoming a vegan. By eschewing the products of cruelty and embracing a life of compassion, you can help heal the rift that we have created between ourselves and other animals. By realizing and acting on the idea that humans have no moral right to inflict suffering on animals for any reason, you will help regain the holism with the Earth and its creatures that humankind has lost.

—HILLARY MORRIS

Try it out! Have fun with it! Don't get too serious or self-righteous once you've done it. Just let it be a joyful and peaceful step in your life! Keep yourself informed about the cruelty in animal agriculture. Even if it means seeing pictures or films of the cruel reality, do it, because it makes it something you have no choice but to act on. Rather than a chore, it becomes part of you.

—RAE SIKORA

People who are nonvegan are living a shadow life, like the people in Plato's allegory who mistake the flickering shadows on the cave wall for reality. I would urge the shadow-watching nonvegans to come into the light and lead a vigorous, full-bodied existence.

—RYNN BERRY

I would ask, if I could do so without the risk of being looked down on as impolite, "What if it were you? Would you like to be someone's food? Or clothing?"

—Narendra Sheth

Whatever you do, please don't tell me that you could never be a vegan. I would rather hear you say that you are trying your best. It may be difficult at first, as it would be to change any habit, but it only gets easier. And one day you might get to the point where you will look back and not be able to remember what life was like before you decided to do what you know is right for yourself. If you knew me before I became vegan, you would know that anyone can do this. I have never felt so fulfilled with any decision I have ever made.

—Alan Epstein

Try it. You'll feel better. The animals will feel better. The Earth will feel better. Talk about your win-win situation!

—Tom Regan

Beyond clean arteries, beyond a heathy body, beyond alleviating animal suffering, to adopt a vegan lifestyle is to become a truly spiritual being. A vegan neither wishes nor inflicts harm upon others. This is a most powerful way of moving through existence, and the ultimate reward is a more peaceful world in which all may live and thrive.

—Michael Klaper

THE VEGAN TABLE

I've found without question that the best way to lead others to a more plant-based diet is by example—to lead with your fork, not your mouth.

—BERNIE WILKE

SUBSTITUTES, ANALOGS, AND OPTIONS

When it comes to making the switch to a vegan diet, most new vegans quite naturally ask what they can use in place of various animal-based foods. As the pace of life in North America continues to spiral faster and faster, many people find they don't have the time or inclination to cook the foods we should all be centering our diets around—pure, wholesome, unadulterated grains, beans, vegetables, fruits, nuts, and seeds. In response to the demand for quick-to-prepare vegan foods that are familiar, meat-free versions of standard North American fare, the natural-products industry has created a slew of meat and dairy analogs. In nearly all U.S. cities and towns, natural-food stores brim with items simulating every conceivable dairy and meat product.

However, it's not sufficiently comforting just to know that these products exist. The fact is, they taste fantastic! Furthermore, there are enough various brands so that if you are dissatisfied with one company's efforts you can try several others until you find the ones you most prefer. There is practically no food that former meat and dairy eaters should feel divested of—there are delicious analogs for truly everything.

What's even better is that vegan substitutes have no cholesterol, and many are low in fat or totally fat free. For some vegans, analogs are transition foods, used to help ease the passage to a radically new way of eating. For others, analogs are dietary staples that bring pleasure and excitement to vegan meals in an aura of familiarity.

VEGAN VERSUS KOSHER

Vegan foods are often the same as pareve kosher foods (those classified as neutral according to Jewish dietary laws—i.e., containing neither meat nor dairy), but these terms are in no way synonymous, and many items that are considered pareve are not acceptable to vegans. For instance, according to kosher standards, eggs, fish, and fish products are not considered animal-based. Even marshmallows made from gelatin *may* be considered pareve because the animal products used in the making of the gelatin have been so altered in the manufacturing process that the definition of *meat,* according to kosher interpretation, no longer applies.

Kosher symbols are also not indicative of the ethicalness, purity, healthfulness, or wholesomeness of a product. They are designed to certify that (1) the animals used in the manufacture of a particular product were slaughtered by ritual standards, and (2) meat and dairy products have not intermingled in any way during processing. The primary purpose of certifying products kosher is to keep meat and dairy products separate so that they are not consumed at the same meal. The mission is not to discourage their consumption altogether.

If you purchase a product labeled kosher, it may likely require further examination to ensure that it is vegan. When necessary, contact manufacturers personally to inquire about specific ingredients. Many have toll-free numbers direct to their customer-service departments. Let them know that for vegans, the origin of the ingredient is vital, and that honey, eggs, fish, and *any* products derived from animals—regardless of how extensively processed they may be—are simply not acceptable.

DAIRY PRODUCTS MINUS THE MOO

The most formidable challenge was giving up cheese—especially really pungent, powerful cheeses. I could eat cheese by the pound! I thought the absolutely perfect meal was a loaf of freshly baked French bread, a bottle of red wine (a Bordeaux, preferably), and big chunks of something like a Stilton or a Brie so ripe it smelled like stinking feet. That was heaven.

—TOM REGAN

For most people intent on becoming vegan, eliminating cow's milk and dairy products is viewed as the final, most difficult and forbidding dietary hurdle. But vegans need not feel deprived. Natural-foods manufacturers have created a smorgasbord of alternatives that rival the taste and versatility of cow's milk and other dairy foods. In addition, many delicious and healthful dairy-free substitutes can be created at home. My books *Vegan Vittles, The Nutritional Yeast Cookbook,* and *The Uncheese Cookbook* are packed with recipes for dairy substitutes (plus hundreds of other vegan recipes) that are quick and easy to prepare and use common kitchen ingredients. Consequently, once someone makes the decision to eliminate dairy products from her or his diet, the only real challenge left is sifting through the vast options at hand, sufficient to satisfy almost any requirement or taste.

Although soft cheese products have been easy to veganize, hard cheese has been one of the most challenging foods for manufacturers to simulate. Many of the "dairy-free" hard-cheese analogs, especially those designed to melt, contain casein, the protein in cow's milk, rendering them nonvegan. Casein is added to these imitation cheeses to achieve the stretchy quality consumers have come to expect of melted dairy cheese. Therefore, inspect labels carefully when looking for a commercially prepared cheese substitute. Casein may also be listed as caseinate, calcium caseinate, or sodium caseinate. Bearing in mind that vegan cheeses do not contain casein and therefore will not melt like dairy-based cheeses, vegans basically have two choices when it comes to cheese substitutes: (1) look for totally vegan cheese analogs (usually in the deli case of natural-food stores), or (2) make your own cheese substitutes at home, using recipes from *Vegan Vittles, The Nutritional Yeast Cookbook,* and/or *The Uncheese Cookbook.*

When converting traditional recipes that call for dairy products to vegan versions, strive for consistency in flavorings. For instance, use plain or unsweetened nondairy milks for savory recipes and sweetened or vanilla-flavored products for desserts. Different brands of products will yield different results. Let personal preference and product availability guide your choice.

Following are suggestions for commercial and homemade replacements for dairy products. As with most substitutes, experimentation will be the best teacher.

Plant Milks

- *Soymilk* can be prepared at home but, in general, it is time-consuming to make, and the homemade versions tend to have a strong, beany flavor and aftertaste. Commercially prepared soymilk is widely available in ready-to-drink liquids. It can be found fresh in cartons in the refrigerator case of natural food stores and supermarkets or in aseptic packages that do not require refrigeration until they are opened. Soymilk can also be blended from commercial powders and instant mixes, allowing the cook to prepare it as needed. Soymilk is available plain, sweetened, or flavored (e.g. vanilla, chocolate, carob, almond, etc.) in regular, low-fat, and fortified versions that can contain added calcium, vitamin B_{12}, and vitamin D. In cooking, soymilk lends a rich, creamy consistency that thickens well but may curdle at high temperatures. Flavors vary among manufacturers, so try different brands to find the ones you like best. Cartons of fresh soymilk will be stamped with a freshness date and should be stored in the refrigerator. Unopened aseptically packaged soymilk will also be stamped with a freshness date, and the unopened package can be stored for several months at room temperature. Opened packages of soymilk and reconstituted powders will stay fresh for three to ten days in the refrigerator.

- *Rice milk* is available fresh and in aseptic packages in varieties and flavors similar to soymilk. Often sweeter, thinner in consistency, and lighter in taste than soymilk, rice milk makes an excellent beverage or cereal topper and, in cooking, is best suited to baked goods, curries, and lighter cream soups and sauces. Opened packages will keep for about a week in the refrigerator.

- *Nut milk* made from almonds is available in aseptic packages. Nut milk may also be prepared at home from "raw" blanched nuts or seeds (unroasted, unsalted nuts or seeds with skins and shells removed) blended with water. Almost any raw nut, seed, or combination may be used. Nut milks are very versatile and have a rich, sweet flavor, depending on the nut employed. They add depth and body to recipes of all kinds. Nut milks should be stored in the refrigerator and will keep for about a week.

  For homemade nut milk, the standard nut- or seed-to-water ratio is ½ cup raw nuts or seeds to 3½ to 4 cups water. Here is a basic recipe:

  1. Grind the nuts or seeds to a fine powder in an electric seed mill, coffee grinder, or dry blender. Place in a blender with ½ cup almost-boiling water. Process on medium speed to make a smooth, thick cream.
  2. *Gradually* add an additional 3 to 3½ cups almost-boiling water and blend on high until creamy.
  3. Strain the mixture through a very fine mesh strainer or through a colander lined with cheesecloth. Sweeten to taste and flavor with a little vanilla extract (about ¼ to ½ teaspoon), if desired. Chill thoroughly. Shake well before using.

- *Oat milk or mixed-grain milk,* plain or flavored, is typically available in aseptic packages. These milks have a rich, full-bodied flavor, leaning toward the sweeter side. They are naturally low in fat, and their characteristics and usage recommendations are similar to rice milk. Opened packages will keep for about a week in the refrigerator.

Vegan Buttermilk

- 1 cup plain nondairy milk, plus 2 teaspoons lemon juice or vinegar
- ¼ cup silken tofu blended with ¾ cup water, 1 tablespoon lemon juice or vinegar, a pinch of salt, and a little sweetener (optional)

Vegan Cheese

- commercially produced, casein-free, plant-based "cheese" (blocks and slices), "Parmesan," and cream-cheese substitutes
- mashed, water-packed tofu, a little olive oil and salt (for ricotta or cottage cheese)
- smoked tofu (good replacement for provolone and mozzarella)
- oil-cured black olives (adds a sharp, salty flavor reminiscent of Parmesan or Romano)
- nutritional yeast flakes (for an overall cheesy taste)
- sweet white miso (adds saltiness and a cheddary tang)
- any of the cheese substitute recipes found in *Vegan Vittles, The Nutritional Yeast Cookbook,* or *The Uncheese Cookbook,* also by Joanne Stepaniak

Plant Butters for Baking

- Spectrum Spread (a brand-name product made of nonhydrogenated, dairy-free solid vegetable shortening from canola oil and soy protein isolate; found in the refrigerated section of natural-food stores)
- ⅞ cup unrefined canola or corn oil to replace 1 cup of butter in recipes (will not work in some baked goods; unrefined corn oil imparts a rich, buttery flavor)
- fruit purées (such as applesauce, mashed banana, or prune purée) can replace some of the fat in baking

Vegan Spreads for Bread

- fruit butter or preserves
- vegetable butter made from puréed, cooked vegetables
- Spectrum Spread (see "Plant Butters for Baking")
- nut butter (peanut butter, cashew butter, almond butter, etc.)
- seed butter (tahini, sunflower butter, etc.)

- plain or seasoned mustard
- mashed avocado
- egg- and dairy-free mayonnaise (plain or seasoned)

Vegan Yogurt and Sour Cream

- plain soy yogurt (commercially produced)
- soy sour cream (commercially produced)
- silken tofu blended with a small amount of lemon juice, a pinch of salt, and a little sweetener

Vegan Cream and Evaporated Milk

- silken tofu blended with a small amount of water, a tiny pinch of salt, a little sweetener, and a little canola oil (optional)

Vegan Puddings and Custards

- silken tofu blended with sweetener, puréed fresh fruit, soaked dried fruit or fruit preserves, and/or flavorings such as vanilla extract, almond extract, carob, or cocoa powder

Vegan Ice Cream and Popsicles

- dairy-free sherbet, ices, and sorbets (check the ingredient label closely, as some may contain dairy products or whey, a by-product of cheesemaking)
- nondairy frozen ice cream
- frozen fruit-juice sticks
- frozen bananas (peel before freezing; wrap in plastic wrap or place in an airtight container)

EGG-FREE COOKING AND BAKING

Eggs are used as binders and thickeners in casseroles and as binders and leavening agents in baked goods. A popular, totally egg-free egg replacer is marketed by Ener-G Foods and sold in natural-food stores and many supermarkets. This powdered egg-replacer consists of a variety of vegetable starches and must be beaten with a liquid before using. It is best used in baked goods only.

Most cookies, baked goods, pancakes, etc., which do not require a great deal of leavening and call for only one egg, can easily be made without the egg. Just be sure to add 2 or 3 extra tablespoons of liquid to the batter. If you feel you need an egg substitute in a recipe, first determine the attribute you are seeking. The following lists present a variety of ingredients and blends to use in recipes in place of eggs. Some of these alternatives, such as nut butter or tomato paste, may affect the flavor or color of your finished product. Let the type of recipe you are preparing and the outcome you desire guide your selection and the quantity you need to use.

To Bind or Thicken Without Eggs

(These are good choices to use when preparing veggie burgers, bean and grain loaves, or casseroles.)

- arrowroot powder
- potato starch
- cornstarch
- oat flour
- soy flour
- garbanzo (chickpea) flour
- whole-wheat flour or unbleached wheat flour
- rolled oats (quick or old-fashioned)
- cooked oatmeal
- cracker meal
- matzo meal
- bread crumbs
- crushed cornflakes
- instant potato flakes
- mashed potatoes
- mashed sweet potatoes
- mashed or blended cooked vegetables
- seed butters (tahini, sunflower butter, etc.)
- nut butters (peanut butter, cashew butter, almond butter, etc.)
- tomato paste

- white sauce (made with nondairy milk)
- soft tofu blended with flour (use 1 tablespoon flour to ¼ cup tofu)

To Lighten Baked Goods Without Eggs

(Each suggestion is equivalent to one egg.)

- 1 tablespoon finely ground flaxseed blended with 3 tablespoons water until frothy and viscous, about 30 seconds. Be sure to grind the flaxseeds in a seed mill or dry blender *before* blending with the water. This is my preferred egg substitute for baked goods. (Flaxseeds are highly perishable and should be stored in the freezer to prevent rancidity.)
- ⅛ pound (¼ cup) soft tofu blended with the liquid called for in the recipe
- 1 heaping tablespoon soy flour or garbanzo (chickpea) flour beaten with 1 tablespoon water
- 2 tablespoons flour, 1½ teaspoons canola oil, and ½ teaspoon nonaluminum, double-acting baking powder beaten with 2 tablespoons water
- 1 teaspoon Ener-G Egg Replacer beaten with 2 tablespoons water
- 1 tablespoon cornstarch and 1 tablespoon instant soymilk powder beaten with 2 tablespoons water
- ¼ cup mashed banana or applesauce and ½ teaspoon nonaluminum, double-acting baking powder

For Eggy Flavor or Color Without Eggs

- nutritional yeast (for flavor)
- vegan chicken-flavored instant broth powder (for flavor)
- tiny pinch of turmeric (for color)
- small amount of prepared mustard (for color)

For the Texture of Cooked Eggs Without Eggs

- crumbled silken or soft regular tofu plain or tossed with any of the "eggy" flavor or color suggestions above
- mashed garbanzo beans (chickpeas) or white beans plain or tossed with any of the "eggy" flavor or color suggestions above

HOW SWEET IT IS

About half the white table sugar manufactured in the United States is cane sugar; the other half is beet sugar. The primary distinction between them, other than being derived from different plants, is the processing method. During the final purification process, cane sugar is filtered through activated carbon (i.e. charcoal), which may be of animal or plant origin. This step is unnecessary for beet sugar and therefore is never done.

Approximately half the cane refineries in the United States use bone char (i.e. charcoal made from animal bones) as their activated carbon source. The bone char used in this filtering process does *not* become part of the finished product and, because it is so far removed from the original animal source, cane sugar processed in this method is deemed kosher pareve. Some vegans prefer to avoid white table sugar altogether rather than chance using a product that was filtered through bone char. Others feel this is picayune and draws inordinate attention to a relatively insignificant aspect of vegan living.

Keep in mind that sugarcane is generally heavily treated with pesticides, and workers on sugar plantations typically earn minimal pay, withstand brutal and often debasing working conditions, and rarely receive benefits. From a vegan perspective, the question of whether or not to use sugar should perhaps hinge more on issues of human suffering, exploitation, and environmental degradation than on minimal amounts of bone char, which may or may not be used in processing.

If you want to use white sugar but prefer to avoid products that may have been processed with bone char, look for beet sugar. It is frequently available in natural-food stores. There is no difference in taste, color, or functionality between beet and cane sugars. Other vegan sugars that may be substituted measure-for-measure for white table sugar include unbleached cane sugar (e.g., turbinado sugar or brand names such as Sucanat or Florida's Crystals), maple sugar, palm sugar (available in Indian markets), date sugar (made from pulverized dates; it's tasty but does not dissolve well), and granular FruitSource (a brand-name sweetener made from granulated grape-juice concentrate and brown-rice syrup), among others.

HONEY BE GONE

There are many natural liquid sweeteners that make ideal vegan alternatives to honey. They are widely available in natural-food stores and some supermarkets. When using them as substitutes in recipes, keep in mind their individual sweetening power. The sweetness of these products can vary significantly from honey, which is about 20 percent or more sweeter than sugar. Also, many natural liquid sweeteners vary in viscosity from thin to very thick.

As a broad guideline, light molasses and rice syrup are about half as sweet as honey. Malt syrups, corn syrup, and dark molasses are only a fraction as sweet as honey. Frozen fruit-juice concentrates, concentrated fruit-juice syrups, and sorghum syrup can range from half as sweet to nearly as sweet as honey. Pure maple syrup and liquid FruitSource (the brand name for a product made from grape-juice concentrate and whole-rice syrup) typically can replace the sweetening power and consistency of honey measure-for-measure in recipes. These two are among the most reliable substitutes in recipes that call for a large quantity of honey and depend on an exact ratio of liquid-to-dry ingredients for a proper outcome, such as cakes and other baked goods.

Following are some tips for using natural liquid sweeteners:

- To replace white sugar with a natural liquid sweetener, reduce the total amount of other liquid ingredients in the recipe by about ¼ cup for each cup of liquid sweetener used.
- To liquefy sweetener that has crystallized (e.g. malt syrup or sorghum syrup), place the jar in a pan of hot water for several minutes.
- To accurately measure liquid sweeteners and keep them from sticking to the measuring utensil, first rub some oil in your measuring cup or on your measuring spoon.

Substitute the following liquid sweeteners for the sweetening power of 1 cup white sugar. Some experimenting may be necessary to achieve the desired results.

- 1 to 1⅓ cups malt syrup
- 1 to 1⅓ cups brown rice syrup
- ½ to ¾ cup pure maple syrup
- ½ cup light molasses
- ½ cup sorghum syrup

INNOVATIVE MEAL PLANNING

The vegan diet lends itself naturally to creativity and experimentation. The beauty of this style of eating is its adaptability to varying schedules, tastes, and levels of cooking ability. Following are a few ideas to help you explore some of the endless possibilities a vegan diet affords.

Salad Meals

Salad meals consist of lettuce and/or other raw or cooked vegetables. For a more substantial meal, combine them with potatoes, grains, pasta, beans, tempeh, or tofu. Salad entrées may be served warm or chilled, plain, tossed with an optional dressing, or served with a dressing on the side.

Soup Meals

A hearty bean-, grain-, or vegetable-based soup makes a satisfying main course, especially when complemented with a whole-grain bread and perhaps a leafy green salad. Cold soups or thin soups make excellent summer fare, whereas thicker soups, stews, and chowders are ideal for colder weather.

Potato Meals

Baked or steamed potatoes smothered with steamed or sautéed vegetables, a vegan gravy, tomato sauce, tofu-based sour cream, or whatever topping strikes your fancy are an easy, fun, and filling entrée any time of the year.

Grain or Pasta Meals

Cook any grain (rice, bulgur, couscous, quinoa, millet, polenta, etc.) or pasta you prefer and top or toss it with a vegan cream sauce, nut-based sauce, tomato sauce, vegetable-based sauce, or just a little olive oil. If desired, add steamed, sautéed, or grilled vegetables, grated raw vegetables, fresh herbs, cooked beans, tofu, or tempeh.

Vegetable Meals

Prepare three to six vegetables using your favorite method (steam, sauté or stir-fry, bake, broil, or grill). For a more substantial meal, include a potato, grain, winter squash, cooked beans, and/or whole-grain bread. Vegetable meals are delicious and interesting, with an abundance of visual appeal. Select organically grown seasonal vegetables whenever possible.

Sandwich Meals

Almost anything that can be put on a bun, a bagel, or an English muffin; layered between two slices of bread; stuffed in a pita pocket; piled on a corn tortilla; or rolled in a flour tortilla or chapati can be called a meal. Grilled vegetables, seasoned tofu, marinated artichoke hearts, sautéed mushrooms, roasted red peppers, grated vegetables, bean pâtés, grain pâtés, salad greens, steamed greens, avocado, tomato, nut and seed butters, veggie burgers, meat analogs—if you can imagine it, it can happen! Sandwich meals are creative, quick, and fun, and the possibilities are endless!

Pizza Meals

Top frozen pizza shells, crusty Italian or French bread (sliced in half lengthwise and widthwise), split English muffins, or pita rounds with homemade or jarred pizza or tomato sauce (cheese-free) and finely chopped vegetables of your choice. Drizzle with a little olive oil and top with a sprinkling of nutritional yeast flakes or vegan Parmesan-cheese substitute and bake in a hot oven until golden brown and crisp.

Ethnic Meals

Nearly all ethnic cuisines feature a variety of vegan specialties you can make from scratch at home, buy at natural food stores (fresh in the deli case or frozen), or order at restaurants. From Middle Eastern falafel and dips, to Indian and Thai curries, to Mexican burritos and beans, to exotic Ethiopian delights, to Italian pasta specialties, to Chinese stir-frys, and on and on—you're bound to find endless options to make "ethnic night" the most anticipated meal of the week.

SECRET INGREDIENTS

It's a challenge to become educated on what food products are vegan and to learn what animal ingredients lurk in foods.

—HOWARD LYMAN

Read food labels closely and look for hidden animal ingredients. It's amazing how frequently animal products are incorporated into so many packaged and processed foods, even those you might never suspect.

Ask about all ingredients in restaurant foods and request to see the label of prepared products if your server is unsure what is in them. Even foods that might on the surface appear vegan (such as stir-frys or rice) are often prepared with chicken broth or beef bouillon. Beans and tortillas frequently contain lard. French fries may be cooked in animal fat. Fresh and dried pastas are often made with eggs. Breads and rolls may include eggs, butter, cow's milk, or whey. Croutons are frequently prepared with butter and/or sprinkled with cheese. Salad dressings and sauces could have cow's milk, sour cream, yogurt, cheese, gelatin, or other nonvegan thickeners added. Soups and gravies may be made with a chicken broth or beef bouillon base or may include cow's milk, cream, yogurt, or eggs. Tomato or marinara sauce could contain meat or meat broth or may have been cooked with animal bones. Even vinaigrette dressings are frequently spiked with Parmesan cheese. Be especially careful at ethnic restaurants because of their use of unfamiliar or more exotic ingredients. For instance, Indian restaurants may use ghee (clarified butter), Middle Eastern restaurants may use laban (yogurt), and Asian restaurants may use fish paste.

Don't be shy about asking questions. The more suppliers become knowledgeable about what is and isn't vegan, the more readily they can comply with requests. Many chefs and food-service workers are surprised to learn about the secret ingredients in foods and are usually quite appreciative when informed.

> *Being more aware about what I buy calls for constant vigilance. It has become very important to know all new or unfamiliar ingredients and processes. For eating at restaurants, I have devised a card that lists all the items I do not want to consume. I give it to the waiter to bring to the chef.*

—Narendra Sheth

Following is a list of common ingredients that are regularly incorporated into a variety of processed foodstuffs. Many of these are exclusively animal-based, others may be animal, vegetable, or synthetically derived. If in doubt, research the origin of the ingredient in question before purchasing or consuming the product, or contact the manufacturer directly. Although this list is far from all inclusive, it will provide a broad-based introduction to some of the mystery ingredients manufacturers put into foods.

Albumin: The protein portion of egg whites, which comprises about 70 percent of the whole. Albumin is also found in animal blood and milk. It is used to thicken, bind, or add texture to processed foods such as cereals, pastries, baked goods, soups, stews, frostings, and puddings.

Anchovies: Small, silvery fish of the herring family. Anchovies are a common ingredient in Worcestershire sauce, Caesar salad, some pizza toppings, and flavor enhancers.

Animal shortening: Fats such as butter, suet, or lard, which are common ingredients in packaged cookies, crackers, snack cakes, refried beans, and other processed foods.

Calcium stearate: A mineral typically derived from cows or hogs. Used as an additive in garlic salt, vanilla extract, vanillin powder, salad-dressing mixes, and meat tenderizers to help blend ingredients or to prevent dry ingredients from caking.

Carmine and cochineal: Also listed as carmine cochineal and carminic acid. A red coloring derived from the ground body of the female cochineal insect and used to color juices, candies, applesauce, ice cream, fruit fillings, baked goods, and other processed foods, as well as some "natural" cosmetics. Unfortunately, it is often not specified on ingredient lists.

Capric acid: Also known as decanoic acid. A component of some animal and vegetable fats. Used to make synthetic flavorings and added to butter, coconut, fruit, liquor, beverages, ice cream, candy, baked goods, and chewing gum. Often not specified on ingredient lists.

Casein: Also listed as caseinate, ammonium caseinate, calcium caseinate, potassium caseinate, or sodium caseinate. An animal milk protein that is added to most commercial cheese substitutes to improve their texture and to help them melt better. It is also added to many dairy products (such as cream cheese, cottage cheese, and sour cream) to make them firmer. Outside the food industry, it is used to make paint, plastic, and glue.

Clarifying agent: Also known as fining agent and clarifier. May be derived from eggs, animal milk, gelatin, fish (see *isinglass,* below), or minerals. It is often used in the filtering process of wine, vinegar, beer, fruit juice, and soft drinks.

Diglycerides: A common food additive derived from animal, vegetable, or synthetic sources. Used in conjunction with monoglycerides, which help emulsify ingredients. Found in commercial baked goods, ice cream, shortening, margarine, peanut butter, beverages, chewing gum, and whipped toppings.

Disodium inosinate: A common flavor enhancer used in canned vegetables and sauce and soup mixes; it may be from animal, fish, vegetable, or fungal sources.

Emulsifiers: Also called surfactants, wetting agents, and surface-acting agents. Derived from cows, hogs, eggs, cow's milk, or vegetable sources, or synthetically produced. This encompasses a large class of food additives (e.g., mono- and diglycerides, lecithin, propylene glycol monostearate, calcium stearoyl-2-lactate, polysorbates 60, 65, and 80, etc.) that help dissimilar ingredients (like oil and water) blend together and stay blended. Found in processed foods, shortening, margarine, peanut butter, ice cream, nondairy creamer, chocolate, commercial baked products, and soft drinks.

Flavor enhancers: A large class of additives derived from meat, fish, or vegetable extracts (e.g., disodium guanylate, monosodium glutamate, disodium inosinate).

Folic acid: Also called folacin and pteroylglutamic acid. A member of the B-vitamin complex, folic acid aids in the formation of red blood cells and is essential for maintaining normal metabolism. Found in liver, yeast, mushrooms, and green leafy vegetables. Used to enrich foods including commercial baked goods, flour, rice, and pasta.

Gelatin: The protein derived from the bones, cartilage, tendons, skin, and other tissue of steer, calves, or pigs. It shows up in many commonplace products, including marshmallows, nonfat yogurts, ice cream, some frosted commercial breakfast cereals, puddings, jelled desserts, frozen desserts, sour cream, some commercial sauces and dressings (including many sold at fast-food restaurants), wine, juice, roasted peanuts, pill capsules, and many hair and nail products. Gelatin labeled "kosher" is sometimes vegan but not always. Vegan gelatin is typically made from a natural sea vegetable called carrageen (also known as Irish moss) and locust bean gum (from the carob tree).

Glycerides (monoglycerides, diglycerides, triglycerides): These emulsifying and defoaming agents, obtained from glycerol found in animal or plant sources, are used in numerous processed foods such as commercial baked goods, peanut butter, shortening, chocolate, whipped toppings, jelly, frozen desserts, margarine, and candy, to preserve, sweeten, emulsify, and improve moisture retention. Outside the food industry, glycerides and glycerol (also known as glycerin and glycerine) are used in the manufacture of cosmetics, perfumes, skin emollients, inks, certain glues and cements, solvents, and automobile antifreeze.

Glycerols: Also known as glycerin and glycerine, and most often used as a component to make glycerides. Glycerols may be animal, vegetable, or synthetic based. Used in jelled desserts, marshmallows, candy, confections, and soft drinks.

Isinglass: A gelatin obtained from fish. Used to clarify alcoholic beverages and in some jelled desserts. (Note: Japanese isinglass is made from agar-agar, a sea vegetable.)

Lactose: This sugar occurs naturally in cow's milk and is also called milk sugar. It is commercially produced from whey and is widely used in the food industry as a culture medium (such as in souring milk), as a humectant, and as an ingredient in a variety of processed products including baby formulas, confections, and other foods. Outside the food industry, it is used in bacteriological media, in pharmacology as a diluent and excipient, and as a medical diuretic and laxative.

Lactic acid: A bitter-tasting acid that is formed (1) by fermenting starch, cow's milk whey, molasses, potatoes, or other foods and neutralizing the acid with calcium or zinc carbonate, then decomposing the result with sulfuric acid, or (2) synthetically by hydrolysis of lactonitrile (vegan). Used to impart a tart flavor, as well as in the preservation of some foods. It occurs naturally in the souring of cow's milk and can be found in dairy products such as cheese and yogurt. It is also used in the production of acid-fermented foods such as pickles, olives, and sauerkraut and is used as an acidulant and flavoring agent in beverages, candy, frozen desserts (including sherbets and ices), chocolate, chewing gum, fruit preserves, and many other processed products. Outside the food industry, it is used chiefly in dyeing and textile printing, and in medicine.

Lanolin: This waxy fat is extracted from sheep's wool and is used in chewing gum, ointments, cosmetics, and waterproof coatings.

Lard: Fat obtained from the abdomen of hogs. Used primarily in baked goods, refried beans, and chewing gum.

Lecithin: Any group of phospholipids occurring naturally in animal and plant tissues and egg yolks. The commercial form of this substance is obtained chiefly from soybeans (although it might sometimes be made from egg yolks, peanuts, or corn). Lecithin is used to emulsify and moisturize food. It can be found in cereal, candy, chocolate, baked goods, margarine, and vegetable-oil sprays. Also used in cosmetics and inks.

Magnesium stearate: An additive used as a preservative or an emulsifier. May be derived from animals (cows, hogs), or mineral or vegetable sources. Found in candy, sugarless chewing gum, and pharmaceutical tablets.

Monoglycerides: A common food additive derived from animal, vegetable, or synthetic sources. Used to emulsify ingredients. Found in commercial baked goods, ice cream, shortening, margarine, peanut butter, beverages, chewing gum, and whipped toppings.

Myristic acid: Also known as tetradecanoic acid. A component of most animal and vegetable fats, although typically derived from cows or sheep. Used in butter, butterscotch, chocolate, some flavorings for beverages, ice cream, candy, jelled desserts, and commercial baked goods. Outside the food industry, it is used in personal-care products.

Natural flavorings: Unless another source is specified on the label, these could include flavorings derived from meat and other animal products. Used to enhance flavor in processed foods, commercial baked goods, beverages, cereals, salad dressings, and condiments.

Oleic acid (oleinic acid): Obtained from animal tallow (see below) and vegetable fats and oil. Used as a defoaming agent and as a synthetic butter, cheese, and spice flavoring agent for baked goods, candy, ice cream and ices, beverages, and condiments. It is widely used as a lubricant and binder in various processed food products and as a component in the manufacture of food additives. Outside the food industry, it is chiefly used in the manufacture of soaps and cosmetics.

Palmitic acid: A component of animal (cows, hogs) and vegetable fats used as an emulsifier. Found in commercial baked goods, and in butter and cheese flavorings.

Pancreatin: Also known as pancreatic extract. A mixture of enzymes used as a digestive aid. Derived from cows or hogs.

Pepsin: An enzyme obtained from the stomachs of pigs. Used as a clotting agent in conjunction with rennet (see below) during the manufacture of cheese and as a digestive ferment in the making of medicines.

Propolis: A resinous cement collected by bees from the buds of trees and used to stop up crevices in and strengthen the cells of hives. Used as a food supplement and an ingredient in some "natural" toothpastes.

Rennet: A coagulating enzyme principally obtained from the stomach lining of calves, kids, pigs, or lambs. Used to curdle cow's milk in foods such as cheese and junket. It may also be used as a firming agent in other dairy products, including cottage cheese, ricotta cheese, sour cream, and cream cheese.

Royal jelly: A substance produced by the glands of bees. Used in some "natural food" preparations and nutrient supplements as a source of B-complex vitamins, minerals, and amino acids.

Sodium stearoyl lactylate: A common food additive used as an emulsifier or a dough conditioner. May be derived from cows, hogs, animal milk, or vegetable-mineral sources. Used in commercial baked goods, cake and pancake mixes, frozen desserts, liquid shortenings, pudding mixes, coffee whiteners, and margarine.

Stearic acid: Also called octadecanoic acid. This is a common fatty acid occurring as the glyceride in tallow (see below) and other animal fats and animal oils. It can also be made synthetically through hydrogenation of oleic acid.

Used in vanilla and butter flavorings, chewing gum, baked goods, butter, beverages, and candy, as well as in the manufacture of soaps, ointments, stearates, candles, cosmetics, medicinal suppositories, and pill coatings.

Suet: The hard white fat found around the kidneys and loins of sheep and cattle. Used commercially in margarine, mincemeats, and pastries. Also used to make tallow (see below).

Tallow: The solid fat of sheep and cattle separated from the fibrous and membranous matter that is naturally mixed with it. Used in margarines and waxed paper. Outside the food industry, it is used in soaps, candlemaking, crayons, rubber, and cosmetics.

Vitamin A (vitamin A_1, retinol): A yellow, fat-soluble vitamin obtained from carotene, which occurs in green and yellow vegetables but may also come from egg yolks or fish-liver oil. Vitamin A is used as a vitamin supplement and to fortify processed foods. Also used as a colorant and preservative in "natural" cosmetics.

Vitamin A_2: A yellow fat-soluble vitamin obtained from fish-liver oil. Vitamin A palmitate is made by reacting vitamin A_2 with palmitic acid, which is obtained from palm oil (derived from palm trees). Vitamin A_2 is used as a vitamin supplement and to fortify processed foods.

Vitamin D: Any of several fat-soluble, antirachitic vitamins (D_1, D_2, D_3). Vitamin D is readily made by the human body upon moderate exposure to sunlight. (Some people, such as darker-skinned and older people and those living in smoggy or cloudy areas, may have a harder time manufacturing vitamin D.) Vitamin D_2 (ergocalciferol) is obtained by irradiating provitamin D (from plants or yeast) with ultraviolet light. Vitamin D_3 (cholecalciferol) is derived from fish-liver oils and sometimes lanolin (sheep's wool fat). Used as a vitamin supplement and to fortify processed foods.

Whey: The watery liquid that separates from the solids in cheesemaking. It is found in crackers, breads, cakes, and a great many other processed foods.

VEGAN NUTRITION

BY VIRGINIA MESSINA, M.P.H., R.D

You are what you eat.

—AMERICAN PROVERB

HEALTH BENEFITS OF VEGAN DIETS

Vegan diets offer clear advantages over standard Western diets. While we are a long way from being able to define the optimal eating plan, it is clear that people who base their diets on plant foods have a lower risk for certain conditions, including some types of cancer, heart disease, diabetes, obesity, hypertension, gallstones, and kidney stones. There are a number of factors related to plant-based diets that may contribute to this protection. Here are some of the most compelling considerations:

- Vegans tend to eat less fat than both omnivores and lacto-ovo vegetarians. Excess fat in the diet may contribute to obesity and raise the risk of cancer. Most important, vegans consume very little saturated fat and *no* cholesterol, since cholesterol is found only in animal foods. This is most likely the primary reason for their lower cholesterol levels and reduced heart-disease risk.

- Vegans consume as much as four times more fiber than omnivores. Fiber protects against colon disease and is an important factor in the reduced rates of colon cancer seen in vegetarians. It also may help to protect against heart disease and diabetes. Fiber is found *only* in plant foods.

- Vegans consume generous amounts of antioxidants. These are components in plant foods (they include certain vitamins, minerals, and non-nutrient components) that protect cells from the damage caused by free radicals. Free radicals are a normal by-product of metabolism, but they play a critical role in the development of cancer and heart disease and perhaps other diseases, like arthritis.

- Vegans eat less total protein than omnivores and lacto-ovo vegetarians and, of course, they eat no animal protein. Animal protein may contribute to higher blood-cholesterol levels and increase the risk of kidney damage; it may also affect bone health.

- Vegan diets are high in phytochemicals, which are found *only* in plant foods. They aren't actually nutrients—that is, we don't need them to live—but they do have important biological properties that can affect health in a myriad of ways. There are hundreds of phytochemicals in a variety of plant foods including vegetables, fruits, grains, nuts, seeds, and legumes.

- Vegans have high intakes of the B vitamin folate. High levels of folate reduce the blood levels of an amino acid called homocysteine. Homocysteine is an independent risk factor for heart disease. Therefore, this may be one important protective factor for vegans.

Given what we know about how vegans eat, we shouldn't be too surprised by their better health profile. All these factors in plant foods combine to provide protection against a number of chronic conditions.

Atherosclerosis and Heart Disease

Atherosclerosis is the buildup of fatty deposits (called plaques) in the arteries. This buildup can impede blood flow to organs, and if arteries leading to the heart are involved, the result can be a heart attack. Other organs can be affected as well, since atherosclerosis also affects blood flow to the kidneys, brain, and other parts of the body.

High blood cholesterol increases the risk of atherosclerosis; the risk is further raised when the cholesterol is oxidized. Diets low in saturated fat and cholesterol and high in antioxidants lower the risk of atherosclerosis. Fiber-rich diets may be protective as well. There is some evidence that high animal-protein intake, too much iron, and low levels of the B vitamin folate also raise the risk. It is no surprise that vegans have a comparatively low risk for heart disease and that they are at even lower risk than other vegetarians. Vegans have lower blood-cholesterol levels because they eat less saturated fat and no cholesterol. Their diets are also rich in antioxidants, fiber, and folate and lower in iron and protein.

Cancer

While there is little evidence that vegans specifically have a lower risk of cancer, the evidence from populations throughout the world is that plant-based diets reduce risk for certain types of cancer. There are many ways that diet might affect cancer risk. Dietary fiber can aid the body in excreting some carcinogens, which are compounds that initiate the cancer process. Promoters, like dietary fat, can prompt cancer cells to divide, setting tumor growth in motion. Also, many enzymes in the body that deactivate carcinogens are themselves increased by phytochemicals in plant foods.

A variety of lifestyle factors afford protection against cancer, and a plant-based diet is among them. This is especially evident regarding colon cancer. The entire environment of the colon is significantly different between meat eaters and those who eat mostly plant foods. Vegetarians have a much lower risk of colon cancer.

The picture for breast cancer is a bit murkier. Worldwide, populations that eat plant-based diets have lower rates of breast cancer. Plant diets produce changes that seem to protect against breast cancer. For example, high blood estrogen raises breast-cancer risk. Some studies show that vegetarian women have lower estrogen levels, perhaps because they eat more fiber and less fat. Despite this, there is no reported difference in cancer rates between vegetarians and nonvegetarians. This may be because most studies have involved Seventh-day Adventist vegetarians whose diets are mostly lacto-ovo and not significantly lower in fat. Studies of vegans might provide a different outcome, but we don't have those data yet.

Hypertension

It is well established that vegetarians have lower blood pressures than omnivores, and there is evidence that vegans have lower blood pressures compared to other vegetarians. The reasons for this are poorly understood since it doesn't seem to be related to sodium intake or body weight, both of which are closely related to blood pressure. There are probably a number of factors in plant foods that help reduce blood pressure.

Kidney Disease

Each day, the kidneys filter the entire volume of blood in the body about sixty times in order to sift out and excrete unwanted chemicals. Diets high in protein force the kidneys to work harder by increasing the rate at which they filter blood. In turn, this places stress on the kidneys and can raise the risk of kidney problems in older people or in people already at risk for kidney disease. Not surprisingly, the filtration rate of the kidneys is lower in vegans than in both lacto-ovo vegetarians and omnivores—presumably because their diets are lower in protein. High cholesterol levels can also contribute to kidney disease, so the lower cholesterol levels of vegans might be protective.

Kidney Stones

Although high calcium intake seems to protect against kidney-stone formation, vegans—whose calcium intake is relatively low compared with other groups—have a lower risk for this condition than omnivores. This may be because their diet is also lower in protein. Excess protein raises rates of calcium excretion which can lead to the formation of kidney stones.

Obesity

A number of studies reveal that vegans tend to weigh less and have less body fat than both omnivores and lacto-ovo vegetarians. Most likely, this is due to the lower fat and higher fiber content of vegan diets. Exercise may also be a contributing factor.

All of the preceding information suggests that vegans enjoy some health advantages over omnivores, and in some cases, over lacto-ovo vegetarians as well. But while vegan diets offer protection, this is only true if they are well balanced and nutrient rich. Planning healthful vegan diets isn't difficult—it's just different. However, it does require some attention to a few specific nutrients.

NUTRIENTS OF SPECIAL INTEREST IN VEGAN DIETS

Planning healthful vegan meals requires focusing on nutrients that are occasionally lower in vegan diets. Traditionally, these have been areas of consideration, but it is important not to lose sight of the fact that vegan diets are especially abundant in many nutrients. For example, compared with both other vegetarians and omnivores, vegans have higher intakes of folate, biotin, vitamin C, iron, and magnesium. Vegetarians as a group also consume more vitamin A (as beta carotene), vitamin E, copper, potassium, and manganese.

However, there is no such thing as the ideal diet that will guarantee adequate nutrient intake for every individual. No matter how you choose to eat, you need to pay some attention to food choices. This is true of omnivore, lacto-ovo vegetarian, and vegan diets. You can easily meet your nutrient needs on a vegan diet provided you shift your focus in meal planning and emphasize certain foods and food groups. Giving up meat and dairy products and filling the empty spots on your plate with whatever you like will not automatically do the trick.

Protein

There is no reason to be concerned about protein, since even on vegan diets there is little risk of deficiency. Plant foods such as grains, legumes, nuts, and seeds are all high in protein. Soy products (such as tofu) are especially rich in high-quality protein; vegetables provide smaller amounts of protein.

The issue of protein quality has received a great deal of attention in the past. This concept has to do with the amino-acid makeup of proteins. Amino acids are the building blocks of protein; foods contain varying arrangements of twenty-two different amino acids. Humans use amino acids from food to create new proteins that the body requires such as enzymes, hormones, and muscle tissue. The human body can actually manufacture many of these amino acids provided it has the raw materials. Nine of the amino acids, however, are dietary essentials since the body cannot make them.

Plant foods like grains, legumes, nuts, seeds, and vegetables do contain all nine of the essential amino acids. Nevertheless, plant proteins are slightly lower in quality than animal proteins because they are not as well digested and their amino-acid patterns are a slightly poorer match to our bodies' needs. All this means is that vegans need to eat more of them. Vegans have a somewhat higher protein requirement than omnivores and perhaps lacto-ovo vegetarians as well. This might seem worrisome since vegans also consume less protein than these other groups, but in fact it isn't a problem at all. Even with higher needs and lower intake, vegans appear to have no difficulty meeting protein needs. The old rules about carefully combining proteins have fallen by the wayside. As long as you eat a variety of plant foods throughout the day and you eat enough whole plant foods to meet your calorie needs, you will achieve adequate protein intake.

Calcium

The calcium requirement for vegans is still undetermined and remains a point of much discussion. Many dietary and lifestyle factors affect calcium requirements, so vegans, especially those who lead active, healthy lifestyles, may actually have lower needs. One dietary factor that appears to affect the way calcium is used is protein. Diets high in protein may increase calcium needs, because protein causes more calcium to be excreted from the body. This is particularly true of proteins high in certain amino acids, which includes most animal proteins and grains.

Knowing this, it is tempting to assume that vegans—who have lower protein intakes than both omnivores and lacto-ovo vegetarians—have lower calcium needs. While this may indeed be true, there is no real evidence to show that vegans have significantly lower calcium requirements than other groups. Many factors affect calcium needs, and the extent to which protein impacts those needs is not clear. (See "Calcium Myths" on p. 214.)

Because there is no actual evidence that vegans do well with less calcium, we must assume—for now—that vegans should strive to meet the recommended dietary intakes. There is evidence, however, that the lower calcium intake of some vegan women may impair bone health. Studies show that low calcium intake is associated with poor bone health in vegans just as it is in omnivores.

Does this mean that calcium intake is a problem for vegans? Well, certainly some vegan diets are too low in calcium. Studies reveal that a number of vegan women have calcium intakes that are only 400 to 500 milligrams per day while the recommendations are for 1,000 or more milligrams. Any diet can be calcium poor if it isn't well planned. Many omnivore women do not meet calcium needs either. Regardless of how you eat, you need to make sure that your diet includes plenty of calcium-rich foods.

For a long time, nutritionists believed that calcium from plant foods was not well absorbed. Studies from Purdue University reveal this isn't true. Calcium from many plant foods is very well absorbed—in some cases better than the calcium from cow's milk.

To meet calcium needs, it is a good idea to make frequent use of foods that are very rich in well-absorbed calcium. For example, make it a point to include leafy green vegetables—such as kale and collard, mustard, and turnip greens—in your meals every day. Be generous as well in your use of calcium-set tofu, calcium-fortified soymilk, calcium-fortified orange juice, blackstrap molasses, and vegetarian baked beans. However, don't overlook the contributions of other foods. Many beans and vegetables provide relatively small amounts of calcium to the diet, but regular use of these foods can contribute several hundred milligrams to the daily intake. Every little bit counts.

However you choose to meet needs, do pay attention to calcium. If you think you aren't coming close to meeting the recommendations on most days, consider a dietary supplement.

One other word of caution. Vegan women have lower levels of estrogen in their blood. While this is protective against breast cancer, it may raise the risk of osteoporosis, because estrogen protects the health of bones. So, it is possible that vegan women may need to take extra steps toward building bone strength.

CALCIUM MYTHS

There is a great deal of misunderstanding about the relationship of calcium and protein to bone health in vegans. This is largely due to data that compares the number of hip fractures in different populations.

The number of hip fractures in a population is often used as a measurement to determine the rate of osteoporosis in that population. The assumption is that groups with poor bone health will have more hip fractures. Worldwide, populations that eat predominantly plant-based diets have the lowest rates of hip fracture—despite the fact that they have low intakes of dairy foods and calcium. In fact, where people drink the most cow's milk, hip-fracture rates are highest. Not surprisingly, protein intake is also high in these groups. Looking at these findings, it's easy to assume that too much dietary protein is worse for bone health than too little calcium. In fact, some people have suggested that diets low in calcium are perfectly healthful as long as the diet is low in protein as well. But it isn't that simple.

Hip fracture rates don't always tell the whole story about bone health. In some Asian countries with low hip-fracture rates (and low calcium intakes), bone health is actually poorer. That is, people may not fracture their hips often, but they have poorer bone density and more fractures of other bones. So why don't they break their hips? There are any number of explanations. One of the most critical is that Asians have a particular hip structure that is resistant to breakage. This has nothing to do with diet or bone density; it's purely a genetic phenomenon. Another reason is that many of these populations reside in warmer climates. Without slippery snow and ice to contend with, people are less likely to fall. Finally, physically active lifestyles are the norm in many of these countries, resulting in better balance and strength in old age and therefore fewer falls.

Apparently, there are reasons for the low rates of hip fractures in these groups that have nothing to do with bone health at all. Even where bone health is better and bones are denser, it isn't always reasonable to point to low-protein diets as the cause. Too many other factors clearly affect bone density in different cultures. Physical activity is one of the most important bone protectors. In populations where bone health is better, it is nearly always true that people are more active. They may also consume less protein, but this is likely much less important than exercise. There are genetic influences here as well; for example, people of African descent metabolize calcium differently so that, all other things being equal, they need less calcium to maintain healthy bones.

On the basis of hip-fracture rates, some people have even suggested that cow's milk actually causes poor bone health because it is a high-protein food. Hip fractures are more common where people drink cow's milk, and cow's milk is indeed high in protein. But, as previously stated, hip fractures in fact don't reveal much about bone health—at least in comparisons of different cultures. While diets high in protein may indeed increase calcium losses, what really matters is the total ratio of calcium to protein in a particular food or in the overall diet. High-calcium foods promote healthy bones even if those foods are high in protein.

The bottom line? It is a grave mistake to try to draw conclusions about calcium needs of vegans based on hip-fracture data from around the world. They don't tell us anything about calcium requirements. What they do suggest is that bone health is dependent on many factors; genetics, lifestyle, and diet all matter.

Vitamin B_{12}

For many vegans, vitamin B_{12} is *the* dietary issue. More controversy exists over this nutrient than any other. The short story is this: Vegans need to supplement their diet with vitamin B_{12} or risk deficiency. There is really very little disagreement about this among health professionals with expertise in vegan diets. Even so, questions and misinformation about vitamin B_{12} continue to make the rounds among vegans. Therefore, it is worth looking at this nutrient more closely.

All vitamin B_{12} comes from bacteria. These bacteria live in the soil and in the intestines of animals. The B_{12} they produce gets incorporated into animal tissue and animal products such as milk and eggs. Thus, animal products become a source of B_{12} for humans. Bacteria on the outside of plant foods also produce B_{12}, and theoretically, when these foods are consumed, they can provide humans with B_{12}. Realistically, normal cleaning of food eliminates most of the available B_{12}; consequently, these foods are not a reliable source.

It has been suggested that some plant foods are good sources of B_{12}, most notably sea vegetables, tempeh, and miso. However, they actually contain what are called B_{12} analogs. These are B_{12}-like compounds that have no vitamin activity. In fact, they compete with real vitamin B_{12} for absorption. Relying on these foods for B_{12} can actually raise a vegan's risk of deficiency.

Vitamin B_{12} is also produced by bacteria living in the human intestines and mouth. Unfortunately, this seems to be of little significance. Only very minute amounts appear to be produced in the mouth—probably not enough to make much of a contribution to intake. Of course, the goal of good dental hygiene is to keep the mouth as bacteria-free as possible. You'd have to go quite some time without brushing your teeth to get the dubious benefits of significant bacterial growth. Furthermore, B_{12} seems to be produced too far down in the intestines to do much good. Vitamin B_{12}-producing bacteria live down in our large intestine (colon) while B_{12} is absorbed higher up in the small intestine. It's a long climb for a bacterium.

Most vitamin B_{12} deficiency is actually due to absorption problems that are unrelated to diet. Among vegans, overt B_{12} deficiency is not very common. One reason might be that humans store large amounts of B_{12}. People who have eaten B_{12}-rich diets in the past are likely to have enough in storage to last them several years. Regardless, it is important to be careful about defining B_{12} deficiency, because symptoms can be subtle. They include a host of neurological problems that range from subtle tingling of extremities, to actual loss of sensation or paralysis, to changes in memory. In fact, some of the symptoms commonly attributed to senility in old age are actually believed to be the result of B_{12} deficiency. The early signs of neurological impairment can occur even when blood levels of B_{12} appear normal. Also, high intake of the B vitamin folate can mask the early signs of B_{12} anemia, because folate can compensate for some of the functions of B_{12}. Finally, there are subtle problems associated with low B_{12} intake that don't manifest as deficiency per se but can affect health. For example, when B_{12} intake is low, levels of the amino acid homocysteine can go up, and this is a significant risk factor for heart disease.

While it may be true that acute B_{12} deficiency is not a pervasive public health problem in the vegan population, vegans, as a rule, do have low vitamin B_{12} levels. It is reasonable to expect that these levels will decrease in many vegans over time as B_{12} stores are used up. In addition, as we age, B_{12} is absorbed less efficiently. This can increase the risk of deficiency when diets are low in B_{12} to begin with.

Fortunately, it is easy to meet vitamin B_{12} needs on a vegan diet. Supplements are the simplest way to do this, but vegans can use fortified foods as well. Check labels of breakfast cereals and meat analogs. Certain brands of nutritional yeast, such as Red Star Vegetarian Support Formula (formerly T6635+), are also good sources of vitamin B_{12}.

Some vegans are loathe to believe that they need supplements or fortified foods to meet B_{12} needs. In some cases, this might reflect a desire to believe that vegan diets are natural and sufficient without supplementation. Historically, vegan diets probably were completely adequate, and there is reason to believe that humans were perfectly suited to do without nonvegan food sources of B_{12}. The requirement for vitamin B_{12} is infinitesimal—only 2 micrograms a day, or about 15 millionths of an ounce. In fact, one teaspoon of vitamin B_{12} would meet the needs of nearly one hundred people for the rest of their lives! In addition, our bodies hoard B_{12} by storing any excess and by recycling what is used. The fact that it is saved, combined with the minimal amount required, suggests that we evolved to live healthfully in a B_{12}-poor environment. Without animal foods in the diet, we probably did just fine on the little bits of B_{12} we picked up here and there through contamination of food and water. In many parts of the world, this is still probably sufficient to meet B_{12} needs. Potential problems exist for Western vegans, however, because our food supplies are well sanitized, and contamination with B_{12}-producing bacteria is less likely. Of course, there are many advantages to eating clean food, so any inconvenience over B_{12} is a small price to pay.

Iron

Vegan diets are actually higher in iron than either lacto-ovo vegetarian diets or omnivore diets. Because dairy foods are deficient in iron and may inhibit iron absorption, vegans have an advantage over lacto-ovo vegetarians regarding this nutrient. In the case of plant diets, the issue is not how much iron is in food—there is plenty. Rather, it is a question of how much gets absorbed, since compounds in plant foods inhibit absorption of iron into the bloodstream. There is no doubt that iron from plant foods is less well absorbed than is iron from meat. Even so, vegans appear to be no more likely to be iron deficient than meat eaters.

Vegans do, however, have lower stores of iron in their bodies. Is this a concern? While low iron stores may reduce the risk of heart disease, they may also raise the risk of deficiency in certain circumstances. For now, the conclusion can be made that vegans should have the same attitude toward iron as the general population. That means vegans must pay some attention to this nutrient and be careful to get enough because—for all types of diets, including those that contain meat—lack of iron is the number-one nutrient deficiency in the United States. It is an important public health problem, so make sure you eat plenty of iron-rich foods daily. Include a good source of vitamin C at each meal, too, since this boosts iron absorption.

Vitamin D

Vitamin D has an identity crisis. It's treated like a nutrient, but it really isn't one. It is vital for good health, of course, but the human body can manufacture all that it needs when the skin is exposed to the sun. The problem is that not everyone gets enough sun exposure. Some people need more than others; for example, darker-skinned and older people make vitamin D less efficiently. It is also harder for people to make vitamin D the farther away they live from the equator, or if they reside in a smoggy or cloudy area. In earlier times, when the majority of people lived in warmer areas, wore less clothing, and spent more time outdoors, no doubt vitamin-D deficiency was not a problem. Today, some people need an alternate source of this compound. Very few foods contain natural vitamin D, so the best solution has been to fortify the food supply. Contrary to popular belief, cow's milk is not a good natural source of vitamin D; it is only a good source when it is fortified, as is all cow's milk in the United States.

For vegans, the best option for vitamin D is adequate sun exposure. For light-skinned people, exposing arms and face (without sunscreen) to summertime sun for fifteen to twenty minutes three times a week should be sufficient. If you are dark skinned or live where summers are short or in a smoggy urban area, you may need much more exposure. This is also true for older people. If you suspect that you don't get enough sunlight, a supplement or fortified foods is a good idea. Many brands of soy and rice milk are fortified, as are some breakfast cereals. If you use a supplement, choose one that provides no more than 10 micrograms of vitamin D, since it is toxic in high doses.

Riboflavin

Few plant foods are rich in riboflavin, although many plant foods contain moderate amounts. Including these foods in the diet on a regular basis should provide adequate supplies of riboflavin. Studies show that most vegans come close to meeting recommended intakes for riboflavin. Presently, there is considerable controversy over the actual requirement for this nutrient, and it is possible that the recommendations are too high. Nevertheless, without hard evidence to guide us, it's a good idea to try to meet riboflavin requirements.

Zinc

Zinc deserves some special attention in all diets. The richest sources in standard North American diets are meat and dairy products. Even so, omnivores tend not to consume as much zinc as they should. Although plant foods are generally much lower in zinc, vegetarian intake appears to be comparable to omnivore intake or slightly lower. There isn't much information available on zinc intakes of vegans. What little data exists indicates that, not surprisingly, vegans consume less zinc than other groups. Although compounds in plants can inhibit zinc absorption, overt zinc deficiency is not a common problem among vegans. Nevertheless, vegans must consider the potential effects of marginal deficiencies. These are harder to pinpoint, but they can become important over time. For this reason, consuming plenty of zinc-rich foods is a good idea.

Fat in Vegan Diets

A trend among some vegans has been to consume only foods that are very low in fat. Although such diets have been linked to significant improvements in heart health, it is likely that the lower intake of saturated fat and the total elimination of cholesterol are responsible for this effect.

Keeping fat intake on the low side is a desirable goal. Excessive fat can cause weight gain and may increase cancer risk. But avoiding all high-fat foods and added fats is probably not necessary for good health and may not be wise. Some fats, like the monounsaturated fats found in nuts, olives, olive oil, canola oil, and avocados, appear to have some health benefits. For one, they may lower the risk of heart disease. Very low-fat diets cause decreases in HDL cholesterol, which is the "good" cholesterol that protects against heart disease. Diets that include monounsaturated fats protect against these decreases in HDL. Monounsaturated fats may also be useful in the treatment of diabetes. Traditional plant-based Mediterranean diets, which protect against cancer and heart disease, make generous use of monounsaturated fats.

Very low-fat vegan diets may also be too low in the omega-3 fatty acids. Since the ratio of certain dietary fatty acids is important, it may be valuable to eat less of certain fats and more of others. A healthful goal is to limit added polyunsaturated fats by eating less safflower, sunflower, and corn oil and replace them with sources of the omega-3 fatty acids (flaxseeds, full-fat soy products, walnuts, and canola oil), along with sources of monounsaturated fats.

Aim for a total fat intake that is low to moderate—about 20 to 30 percent of calories—since both excess fat and too little fat seem to have disadvantages.

COW'S MILK: NOT QUITE THE PERFECT FOOD

Dairy consumption is one of the dietary habits that really distinguishes vegans from other vegetarians. Some nutritionists continue to question the adequacy of dairy-free diets because cow's milk has maintained a solid reputation as a dietary essential. Of course, it makes no sense to believe that any one food is crucial to the diet. You need calcium, protein, and riboflavin, but it doesn't matter where you get them as long as you do get them. The bias in Western cultures in favor of cow's milk is based more on habit, economics, and politics than on science. There is a clear ethical rationale for avoiding cow's milk, and as long as calcium can be obtained elsewhere, there is no reason for dairy consumption. However, evidence shows that diets which contain little or no dairy products could have some health advantages as well. Admittedly, the health risks associated with dairy consumption are speculative at best, but when combined, they are worthy of some attention.

Cow's Milk Intolerance

Cow's milk intolerance represents an interesting piece of nutrition history. It involves a decreased ability to digest lactose, the sugar found in milk and some milk products. As people age, they become less efficient at manufacturing the enzyme lactase, which is necessary to digest this sugar. Nutrition anthropologists believe that as recently as ten thousand years ago, no adult humans could digest milk sugar. The enzyme lactase was present in babies so that they could digest their mother's milk. Lactase production slowly decreased throughout childhood and into adulthood as a normal part of development. Approximately ten thousand years ago, a mutation occurred that allowed some adults—namely those living in northern Europe—to continue digesting milk throughout adulthood. Today, many people of northern European descent around the world can digest milk their entire lives. Conversely, many people from other parts of the world—such as those indigenous to southern Europe, the Mideast, Asia, Africa, and the Americas—digest it less well. Symptoms of this intolerance to cow's milk include nausea, gas, and diarrhea. Not surprisingly, cow's milk consumption is lower in parts of the world where lactose intolerance is more common. Lactose intolerance is not a problem per se. Symptoms are avoided when dairy consumption is limited or when people use specially treated milk in which the sugar is predigested. The story of lactose intolerance is an intriguing one since it suggests that cow's milk is a less natural food than most people believe.

Diabetes

A 1991 study in Finland was among the first to suggest that, in certain groups of children, cow's milk consumption in infancy—whether as regular cow's milk or as infant formula made from cow's milk—was associated with greater risk of diabetes later in life. These groups of children produced antibodies to cow's milk protein. The antibodies destroyed cells in the body that produce the essential hormone insulin. Since then, other studies have confirmed this finding, showing that cow's milk consumption throughout childhood could pose a risk in children who were genetically susceptible to this problem. Other studies, however, have not supported these findings.

Ovarian Cancer

One study at Harvard University found that women who consume dairy foods have a higher risk of ovarian cancer. Other studies have not supported this finding. If such a risk exists, it probably involves the sugar galactose, a component of the milk sugar lactose. Galactose itself undergoes breakdown and metabolism. However, some women lack the enzyme for proper metabolism of this sugar. In this case, high blood levels of unmetabolized galactose could possibly damage ovaries.

Anemia

Although cow's milk consumption does not directly influence iron status in most people, overconsumption of dairy foods can be a very real problem in young children. Particularly among toddlers and preschoolers, too much cow's milk in the diet can make a child less hungry for iron-rich foods. Cow's milk doesn't contain iron, and if it displaces other foods, the result is a diet low in iron. In addition, cow's milk can interfere with iron absorption from other foods. The net result is that children who drink too much cow's milk run a risk of iron-deficiency anemia.

Heart Disease

The culprit here, once again, is cow's milk sugar, galactose, which may attach to proteins in the walls of the arteries, promoting the buildup of plaque.

Colic

Colic is an uncomfortable digestive disorder experienced by infants. A sensitivity to cow's milk protein may be one cause. In fact, even in breast-fed infants, colic can occur if cow's milk protein from the mother's diet is passed to the infant through her breast milk.

Vitamin D Toxicity

In the United States, law requires that cow's milk be fortified with vitamin D; each quart must contain 10 micrograms. However, large volumes of cow's milk are fortified simultaneously. As a result, if the milk isn't properly mixed, some quarts on the grocery store shelves may contain virtually no vitamin D while others may have many times the federal requirement. This is cause for concern because vitamin D is toxic in amounts just five times greater than the requirements. In one survey, some samples of cow's milk were found to contain five hundred times more vitamin D than the amount allowed by the federal government.

Cataracts

In certain people, high blood levels of the cow's milk sugar galactose can lead to cataract development. This affects only people who have an impaired ability to metabolize galactose, although this relationship is still somewhat speculative.

VEGAN DIETS THROUGHOUT THE LIFE CYCLE

Well-planned vegan diets are a sound choice for all stages of the life cycle. At certain times of life, however, the need for very nutrient-dense diets is more important than others, and special attention to menu planning becomes necessary for everyone, including vegans. A few guidelines make it easier to plan vegan diets for pregnant women, infants and babies, children and teens, older people, athletes, and diabetics.

Pregnancy

Pregnant women require more of nearly all the essential nutrients. All pregnant women need to eat a nutrient-rich, well-balanced diet. When diets are well balanced, vegan women are as likely as nonvegetarians to have a healthy pregnancy and baby. To ensure the healthiest pregnancy possible, follow these guidelines:

1. *Consume enough food to maintain an ideal weight gain.* It takes about 80,000 calories to build a baby and maintain a healthy pregnancy. Fortunately, these calories can be spread over nine months of meals. For most women, a reasonable weight gain is one to one-and-a-half pounds per week starting with the fourth month of pregnancy. Check with your health-care provider to determine if a different pattern of weight gain is advisable for you, since needs vary.

2. *Limit empty-calorie foods.* With higher caloric requirements, you have room for a few special items. Nevertheless, nutrient needs are a priority as well. A diet based on a wide variety of whole plant foods is the healthful way to eat during pregnancy and is essential for meeting the high nutrient needs of pregnancy.

3. *Consume foods fortified with vitamin B_{12} or take a daily supplement of 2 micrograms.* Even if you are a new vegan and you believe that your body has plenty of stored vitamin B_{12}, the storage supply may not find its way to the fetus.

4. *Eat a very calcium-rich diet.* The requirement for pregnancy is 1,000 to 1,300 milligrams a day, depending on a woman's age. Make it a daily goal to consume leafy green vegetables (at least a cup), calcium-set tofu, and calcium-fortified drinks like fortified rice or soymilk and orange juice. Add blackstrap molasses to dishes. If you think that you might run short on calcium intake, then do take a supplement.

5. *Eat plenty of iron-rich foods.* It's very likely that your health-care provider will prescribe iron supplements for you. They are the norm for all pregnant women. Even so, make it a habit to eat good food sources of iron, such as beans, whole grains, and dried fruit.

6. *Get adequate sun exposure or talk to your health-care provider about a vitamin D supplement.*

Breast-feeding

When women breast-feed, they need to consume a diet that supports their needs as well as the process of manufacturing milk—one that provides enough nutrition for a rapidly growing baby. Not surprisingly, nutrient needs are quite high at this time—in some cases, higher than for pregnancy. Your diet should be similar to the diet you followed during pregnancy except that you need more calories—about 200 more per day—and more fluids. You will need more protein as well, but the extra calories—if they come from whole foods, such as grains, legumes, nuts, and seeds—should provide plenty of the extra protein required. Remember also to continue with vitamin B_{12} supplements or use fortified foods. Get plenty of sun exposure or use vitamin D supplements.

Infants

Guidelines for raising a healthy vegan infant are quite similar to those for omnivore babies. For all babies, the best food for the first year of life is breast milk. There are decided advantages to breast-feeding. Even if you can't or don't want to breast-feed for an entire year, do it for as long as you can. If you choose not to breast-feed, your baby should have a commercial infant formula. In vegan families, soy formula is a good choice. Follow these guidelines for a well-fed vegan infant:

1. Breast milk or soy infant formula is the only food your baby needs for the first four months or so of life. Breast milk is by far the best choice for your baby. If you choose not to breast-feed or if you supplement breast-feedings with formula, purchase a commercial brand of formula. Never make your own formula from soymilk or grains and never give a baby regular soymilk or cow's milk. There is only one best food for an infant, which is breast milk, and one suitable substitute, which is commercial infant formula.

2. Breast-fed infants should have the following supplements:

   - Vitamin B_{12} if the mother's diet is not supplemented.
   - Vitamin D beginning at around three months if the infant doesn't get enough sun exposure.

- Iron supplements beginning at around four months.
- Fluoride (after six months) if the local water supply isn't fluoridated.

3. Begin to introduce solid foods around four months if your baby appears to be ready. Generally, babies are ready for solids if their birth weight has doubled and they demand more than eight feedings a day, can sit up without support, and can hold their head up. All babies should be consuming some solid food by six months. You can take the following steps for feeding solids:

- Introduce one new food at a time and wait two to three days before introducing another food. This will help identify any foods that cause an allergic reaction.
- Begin with an iron-fortified infant cereal, such as rice cereal (it is unlikely to cause allergies). Dilute it well with breast milk or formula and feed just a few teaspoons a day. Then, if this is tolerated well, introduce other cereals, such as iron-fortified oat and barley cereals.
- When your baby is eating one-third to one-half cup of cereal a day in two feedings, begin to introduce mashed fruits and vegetables, again introducing one new food at a time at three-day intervals. Good choices include smooth applesauce, pureed cooked peaches or pears, potatoes, carrots, sweet potatoes, green beans, and raw mashed bananas and avocado.
- At seven to eight months, offer your baby fruit juice from a cup.
- Also at seven to eight months, begin to offer higher protein foods, such as thoroughly cooked and pureed legumes or mashed tofu.
- At ten months, offer your baby finger foods, such as small tofu chunks, crackers, and bread. Frozen bagels are a soothing food for teething babies to gnaw on.
- At one year of age, you can introduce small amounts of smooth nut butters and stronger tasting vegetables like kale (mix it with apple-sauce or blended avocado to sweeten or temper the taste).

4. To keep your baby's diet as healthful as possible, avoid salt and sugar. If you prepare baby foods from canned or frozen fruits and vegetables, choose ones that have no salt or sugar added.

Vegan Children

Healthy babies are enthusiastic eaters; they are hungry because they grow quickly. The guidelines for feeding these littlest vegans are fairly straightforward. As children approach the toddler and preschool years, however, growth slows and children begin to want to have a say in what they eat. Getting them to eat healthful foods can be a challenge. And as they venture out to friends' houses and preschool, they will quickly encounter many nonvegan situations. In planning healthful diets for young children, keep a few basics in mind.

1. Focus on building your child's diet around a variety of whole foods. This may not be possible every day of the week as children can have stubborn food jags and periods when they are simply not hungry. But aim for this as best you can.

2. Children have especially high needs for calcium, zinc, iron, and vitamin D compared with their caloric requirements. They need a diet that is very dense in these nutrients to maintain good health. If you aren't confident that your child eats enough good sources of these foods, a multivitamin and mineral tablet is in order.

3. Young children have small stomachs that fill up quickly, so provide them with frequent small meals. Eating five to six minimeals a day is preferable to three big meals.

4. Make sure your child has a daily source of vitamin B_{12} either from a supplement or from fortified foods.

In many families, children are breast-fed beyond their first year. If toddlers aren't breast-fed, they can have regular, full-fat, calcium-fortified soymilk beginning on their first birthday. Rice milk and nut milks are fine occasionally but are too low in protein for regular use.

As children grow older, their dietary preferences generally expand. Even so, many will turn up their noses at legumes and vegetables. Be sure to introduce a wide variety of foods often and don't make too big a deal about new foods or disliked foods. It is important for children to see parents enjoying many different kinds of food. Here are some suggestions for incorporating variety into your child's diet:

- Offer plenty of easy-to-eat finger foods and raw vegetables (which have a milder taste than cooked ones).
- Let children help with food preparation, and provide them with fun foods like baby vegetables, vegetable kabobs, or salads of raw or cooked vegetables in the shape of animals.
- Sneak rejected foods into well-liked dishes.
- Serve soymilk or soft tofu in puddings, shakes, or fruit smoothies.
- Make pancakes or French toast using fortified soymilk.
- Add tiny pieces of vegetables to soups and stews or spaghetti sauce.
- Add finely chopped vegetables to homemade veggie burgers or muffins.

When planning meals for your vegan child, don't skimp too much on fat. There is no evidence that very low-fat vegan diets are either optimal or safe for children. Higher-fat foods, such as tofu, soymilk, nuts, seeds, nut and seed butters, and avocado, are nutrient-rich choices that should be regular parts of the diet for vegan children. Even small amounts of added fats and oils are fine to include. Remember that variety is the key. Don't emphasize these high-fat foods in your child's diet, but do include them.

Vegan Teens

The teen years are a period of rapid growth, faster than any other time except infancy. Needs for calories, protein, calcium, and, especially for girls, iron, increase dramatically. All teens need guidance when it comes to planning meals and eating well. North American teens in particular tend to have less than optimal diets at a time when good nutrition is crucial.

Information is not yet available regarding the health and growth of vegan teens; however, studies indicate that lacto-ovo vegetarian teens seem to do fine. As with younger children, the key to good health is a diet based on a wide variety of whole foods that emphasizes plenty of calcium, iron, and zinc. Sources of vitamin B_{12} and vitamin D (either via the sun or a supplement) are necessary. Since teens generally have good appetites and tend to eat a lot, they are usually able to get all the calories they need. Nonetheless, it is important to make certain your teen's food choices are the best.

Studies show that teens eat a lot of meals on the go, as snacks and as part of social events. It's no wonder that the average teen tends to frequent local fast food restaurants often. If there is a vegan teen in your house, here are some helpful guidelines:

- Make sure the kitchen is well stocked with a variety of portable meals and snacks.
- Make sure that fast meals that can be prepared at home are available.
- Encourage family dinners as often as possible, since teens who eat with their families tend to have the best nutrient intakes.
- For fast meals, stock the kitchen with vegan muffins, soy yogurt, individual serving sizes of fortified soymilk, cheeseless pizza slices (frozen and ready to pop into the microwave or toaster oven), hummus and pita bread, bagels with nut butters, fruit, pretzels, frozen fruit ices, instant oatmeal, and frozen veggie burgers.

Older Vegans

Older people have special nutritional needs, and this is true for older vegans as well. For example, the ability to absorb vitamin B_{12} decreases with age in many people. If B_{12} stores are already low, decreased absorption can hasten deficiency symptoms. Symptoms of B_{12} deficiency can include memory loss, confusion, and even dementia, so B_{12} deficiency can be misdiagnosed as age-related dementia. Therefore, older vegans need to include a good source of B_{12} in their diets and have B_{12} levels checked regularly. All older people, regardless of diet, should use B_{12} supplements. It also becomes more difficult to manufacture vitamin D, so older people may require increased sun exposure to meet their needs for this nutrient. The recommended intake for calcium for older people is 1,200 milligrams. Many women, regardless of the type of diet they follow, will have difficulty achieving such high intakes without supplements.

By paying attention to these dietary issues, older vegans can obtain all the nutrients they require. Moreover, vegan diets probably offer some real advantages and protection at a time of life when heart disease, kidney problems, and diabetes most often strike.

Many older individuals experience a loss of taste because the number of taste buds actually decreases dramatically with aging. This means that food may not taste as good as it used to. Even though foods taste more bland, don't make the mistake of gravitating toward very salty or highly sweetened items. Instead, perk up flavors by adding dried fruits to hot cereals or lentil dishes or splashing fresh lemon juice or rice vinegar on vegetables. Vegan cooking also offers great opportunities to try spicier cuisine, such as Indian curries and Thai dishes. Using fresh ingredients—especially fresh herbs—can be helpful since their flavor is more intense.

If older vegans suffer from the empty-nest syndrome or the loss of a spouse, it can be hard to get enthused about cooking. But simple and fast can still be healthful and good. Here are some ideas for quick, wholesome, and tasty meals:

- baked potatoes with canned vegetarian beans
- cereal with soymilk and fruit
- fruit smoothies
- instant soup
- whole-grain toast with nut butter and banana slices
- pasta with sauce from a jar
- canned soup with toast
- frozen veggie burgers

You can follow the same general guidelines for healthful eating as outlined in the Vegan Food Pyramid (Appendix A). However, you may need to cut back on calories a bit if weight gain becomes a problem, since many older people need fewer calories.

Vegan Athletes

Because physical activity requires muscle, which is made of protein, it isn't surprising that high-protein foods like meat have long been considered the basis of the athlete's diet. It does take a bit of extra protein to perform endurance exercises, because exercise increases the rate of metabolism of amino acids. It also takes extra protein to build muscles. Yet these increases in protein needs are small and are easily met by vegan diets. For most athletes, they are readily supplied through increased food consumption. Vegan athletes tend to get the extra protein they need without any effort as long as they choose whole plant foods to provide the additional calories they require. Elite, competitive athletes who train rigorously are an exception. Their protein needs could be twice as high as those of nonathletes. In this case, a regular varied vegan diet may not automatically provide the additional protein they require. But don't turn to protein powders or other supplements. Just make an effort to include one or two additional servings of beans or soy products every day. This will easily provide enough protein.

Athletes may also need extra iron because they have greater muscle mass and blood volume, and because iron is lost through sweat. Vegan athletes should make certain they are consuming plenty of iron-rich foods, as well as vitamin C to enhance iron absorption. Female athletes and female vegetarians both have lower iron stores than the general population. Therefore, vegan women athletes should take care to include plenty of iron-rich foods in their diets. But unless true iron deficiency is a problem, it probably isn't a good idea to take supplements.

Some female athletes may also experience amenorrhea (loss of menstruation). This is a relatively common problem among young female athletes in general and may be more prevalent among vegetarian athletes—although at this time data are inconclusive. There is some health risk associated with amenorrhea. It is caused by low blood estrogen levels, which can negatively impact bone health. Even though exercise itself protects bones, women who lose their periods seem to have poorer bone health.

Since lower estrogen levels among vegetarian women are probably due in part to higher fiber and lower fat intakes, one way to counteract this problem is for vegan female athletes to eat somewhat more fat and less fiber than usual. This does not mean that they should eat a fatty, refined diet. It might be a good idea, however, to add some healthier high-fat foods to the diet, like nuts, seeds, avocado, soy products, and small amounts of beneficial oils such as canola and olive oil—and perhaps to occasionally eat some refined foods like pasta. If missed periods are a problem, calcium supplements would be a good idea. Finally, although this may not be an acceptable solution for all athletes, decreased training can help maintain normal menstrual cycles.

Vegan Diets for Diabetes

In the days when typical diabetic diets were high-protein and low-carbohydrate, vegetarianism was taboo. Now, the best approach to controlling diabetes seems to be a diet that is generous in complex carbohydrates, with an emphasis on high-fiber foods, and moderate in protein and fat. Diets for people with diabetes are actually highly individualized. Whatever works to control your blood glucose and to prevent long-term complications is an appropriate diet for you, provided it also meets nutrient needs. For example, some studies show very low-fat diets to be best for controlling diabetes but, in some people, a diet high in monounsaturated fats may actually be ideal.

Because some of the most serious complications of diabetes include atherosclerosis and kidney disease, a vegan diet, which lowers risk for both of these problems, really does make good sense. If you have diabetes and take medication—either oral medication or insulin injections—and you want to adopt a vegan diet, do work closely with your physician and a dietitian. Your physician may need to reduce your medication dosage when you make the change to a vegan diet, and careful monitoring of blood glucose becomes crucial.

When consulting with a dietitian, diabetics should seek out a professional who is familiar with planning well-balanced vegan diets. Traditionally, diets for people with diabetes were based on the exchange lists, which included both meat and dairy products. Although it isn't necessary to use the exchange lists at all, many people find them useful. Exchange lists for vegetarians and vegans are available.

VEGAN NUTRITION CHARTS

FAT INTAKE OF VEGANS, LACTO–OVO VEGETARIANS, OMNIVORES

	Nonvegetarian	Lacto–ovo vegetarian	Vegan
Total fat as percent of calories	34–38%	30–36%	28–33%
Milligrams of cholesterol per day	300–500	150–300	0

DAILY REFERENCE INTAKES

Following are the recommended intakes of nutrients for adult men and women.

mg: milligram
mcg: microgram
RE: retinol equivalent

Nutrient	Males	Females
Biotin	30–100 mcg	30–100 mcg
Calcium	1,000–1,200 mg	1,000–1,200 mg
Chromium	50–200 mcg	50–200 mcg
Copper	1.5–3.0 mcg	1.5–3.0 mcg
Fluoride	3.8 mg	3.1 mg
Folate	200 mcg	180 mcg
Iodine	150 mg	150 mg
Iron	10 mg	15 mg
Magnesium	400–420 mg	310–320 mg
Manganese	2–5 mg	2–5 mg
Molybdenum	75–250 mcg	75–250 mcg
Niacin	19 mg	15 mg
Pantothenic acid	4–7 mg	4–7 mg
Phosphorus	700 mg	580–700 mg
Potassium	1,600–2,000 mg	1,600–2,000 mg
Protein	63 grams	50 grams
Riboflavin	1.7 mg	1.3 mg
Selenium	70 mcg	55 mcg
Sodium	500 mg	500 mg
Thiamin	1.5 mg	1.1 mg
Vitamin A	1,000 RE	800 RE
Vitamin B_6 (Pyridoxine)	2 mg	1.6 mg
Vitamin B_{12}	2 mcg	2 mcg
Vitamin C	60 mg	60 mg
Vitamin D	5–10 mcg	5–10 mcg
Vitamin E	10 mg	8 mg
Vitamin K	80 mcg	65 mcg
Zinc	15 mg	12 mg

CALCIUM CONTENT OF FOODS

Food	Calcium (mg)
Legumes (1 cup cooked)	
Black beans	103
Chickpeas	78
Great northern beans	121
Kidney beans	50
Lentils	37
Lima beans	52
Navy beans	128
Pinto beans	82
Vegetarian baked beans	128
Soy Foods	
Soymilk (1 cup)	84
Soymilk, fortified (1 cup)	250–300
Soy nuts (½ cup)	252
Soybeans (1 cup cooked)	175
Tempeh (½ cup)	77
Tofu (½ cup) *[if made with calcium sulfate]*	120–350
Textured soy protein (½ cup rehydrated)	85
Nuts and Seeds (2 tablespoons)	
Almonds	50
Almond butter	86
Brazil nuts	50
Sesame seeds	176
Tahini	128
Vegetables (½ cup cooked)	
Bok choy	79
Broccoli	89
Butternut squash	42
Collard greens	178
Kale	90
Mustard greens	75
Sweet potato	35
Turnip greens	125

continued on next page

Food	Calcium (mg)
Fruits	
Calcium-fortified orange juice (1 cup)	300
Dried figs (5)	258
Orange	56
Raisins (⅔ cup)	53
Grains	
Corn bread (2-ounce piece)	133
Corn tortilla	53
English muffin	92
Pita bread (1 small pocket)	31
Other Foods	
Blackstrap molasses (1 tablespoon)	187
Rice Dream, fortified (1 cup)	300
Vegelicious (1 cup)	300

VITAMIN B$_{12}$ CONTENT OF FOODS

Note: Fortification of commercial products can change over time, so it is always a good idea to check the label.

Food	B$_{12}$ (mcg)
Breads, Cereals, Grains	
Grapenuts (¼ cup)	1.48
Kelloggs Corn Flakes (¾ cup)	1.50
Nutrigrain (⅔ cup)	1.50
Product 19 (¾ cup)	6.00
Raisin Bran (¾ cup)	1.50
Total (1 cup)	6.20
Meat Analogs	
(Serving sizes are 1 burger or 1 serving according to package)	
Loma Linda "Chicken" Nuggets	3.00
Loma Linda Sizzle Franks	2.00
Morningstar Farms Grillers	6.70
Worthington Stakelets	5.16
Fortified Soymilk / Vegetable Milks	
(Serving is one 8-ounce cup)	
Better Than Milk	0.60
Edensoy Extra	3.00
Soyagen	1.50
Vegelicious	0.60
White Wave Silk	3.00
Other	
Red Star brand Vegetarian Support Formula nutritional yeast flakes (1 tablespoon)	4.00

RIBOFLAVIN CONTENT OF FOODS

Food	Riboflavin (mg)
Bread, Cereals, Grains	
Barley, whole (½ cup)	0.13
Bran flakes (1 cup)	0.60
Cheerios (1¼ cups)	0.42
Corn flakes (1¼ cups)	0.40
Granola (¼ cup)	0.42
Grapenuts (¼ cup)	0.42
Nutrigrain (¾ cup)	0.40
Pasta, enriched (½ cup)	0.18
Pasta, whole wheat (½ cup)	0.03
Pumpernickel bread (1 slice)	0.17
Rice Krispies (1 cup)	0.40
Wheaties (1 cup)	0.42
Vegetables (½ cup cooked)	
Asparagus	0.10
Beet greens	0.21
Collards	0.09
Mushrooms	0.14
Peas	0.12
Spinach	0.17
Sweet potatoes	0.14
Sea Vegetables (½ cup cooked)	
Alaria	2.73
Dulse	1.91
Kelp	2.48
Nori	2.93
Fruit	
Banana	0.11
Legumes (½ cup cooked)	
Kidney beans	0.09
Soybeans	0.24
Split peas	0.09

RIBOFLAVIN CONTENT OF FOODS *continued*

Food	Riboflavin (mg)
Soy/Vegetable Milks (1 cup)	
Edensoy	0.06
Edensoy Extra	0.10
Soyagen	0.17
Vegelicious	0.17
Vitasoy Original	0.17
Westsoy Plus	0.42
Nuts/Seeds (2 tablespoons)	
Almonds	0.25
Almond butter	0.19
Peanuts	0.12

VITAMIN D CONTENT OF FOODS

Food	Vitamin D (mcg)
Cereals, Grains	
Bran flakes (1 cup)	1.83
Corn flakes (1 cup)	1.83
Granola (¼ cup)	1.83
Grapenuts (¼ cup)	2.40
Fortified Soymilk or Vegetable Milk (1 cup)	
Edensoy Extra	1.00
Rice Dream	2.50
Vegelicious	1.00
Vitamite	2.50
Westsoy	2.50

IRON CONTENT OF FOODS

Food	Iron (mg)
Breads, Cereals, Grains	
Barley, whole (½ cup cooked)	1.60
Bran flakes (1 cup)	11.0
Bread, whole wheat (1 slice)	0.86
Bread, white (1 slice)	0.68
Cream of Wheat (½ cup)	5.50
Oatmeal, instant (1 packet)	6.30
Pasta, enriched (½ cup cooked)	1.19
Rice, brown (½ cup cooked)	0.50
Wheat germ (2 tablespoons)	1.20
Vegetables (½ cup cooked unless otherwise indicated)	
Acorn squash	0.90
Avocado (½ raw)	1.00
Beet greens	1.38
Brussels sprouts	0.90
Collards	0.90
Peas	1.20
Pumpkin	1.70
Spinach	1.50
Swiss chard	1.90
Tomato juice (1 cup)	1.30
Turnip greens	1.50
Sea Vegetables (½ cup cooked)	
Alaria	18.10
Dulse	33.10
Kelp	42.00
Nori	20.90
Fruits	
Apricots (¼ cup dried)	1.50
Prunes (¼ cup)	0.90
Prune juice (½ cup)	1.50
Raisins (¼ cup)	1.10

Food	Iron (mg)
Legumes (½ cup cooked)	
Baked beans, vegetarian	0.74
Black beans	1.80
Chickpeas	3.40
Kidney beans	1.50
Lentils	3.20
Limas	2.20
Navy beans	2.50
Pintos	2.20
Soybeans	4.40
Split peas	1.70
Tempeh	1.80
Tofu	6.60
Textured soy protein (½ cup rehydrated)	2.00
Soymilk	
Soymilk (1 cup)	1.80
Nuts/Seeds (2 tablespoons)	
Cashews	1.00
Pumpkin seeds	2.50
Sunflower seeds	1.20
Tahini	1.20
Other Foods	
Blackstrap molasses (1 tablespoon)	3.30

ZINC CONTENT OF FOODS

Food	Zinc (mg)
Bread, Cereals, Grains	
Barley, whole (½ cup cooked)	1.20
Bran flakes (1 cup)	5.00
Granola (¼ cup)	0.71
Grapenuts (¼ cup)	1.20
Millet (½ cup cooked)	0.42
Nutrigrain (¾ cup)	3.70
Oatmeal, instant (1 packet)	1.00
Shredded wheat (1 ounce)	0.93
Special K (1⅓ cups)	3.70
Wheat germ (2 tablespoons)	2.30
Vegetables (½ cup cooked)	
Asparagus	0.43
Collards	0.61
Corn	0.87
Mushrooms	0.68
Okra	0.57
Peas	0.95
Potato	0.44
Spinach	0.69
Sea Vegetables (½ cup cooked)	
Irish moss	1.95
Kelp	1.23
Nori	1.05
Legumes (½ cup cooked)	
Aduki beans	2.00
Black–eyed peas	1.10
Chickpeas	1.30
Cranberry beans	1.00
Hyacinth beans	2.70
Kidney beans	0.95
Lentils	1.20
Lima beans	0.95
Navy beans	0.90

Food	Zinc (mg)
Legumes *continued*	
Pinto beans	0.90
Soybeans	1.00
Split peas	1.00
Tempeh	1.50
Tofu	1.00
TVP	1.37
Nuts/Seeds (2 tablespoons)	
Brazil nuts	1.30
Cashews	0.96
Peanut butter	1.00
Peanuts	1.80
Pumpkin/squash seeds	1.20
Sunflower seeds	0.90
Tahini	1.30

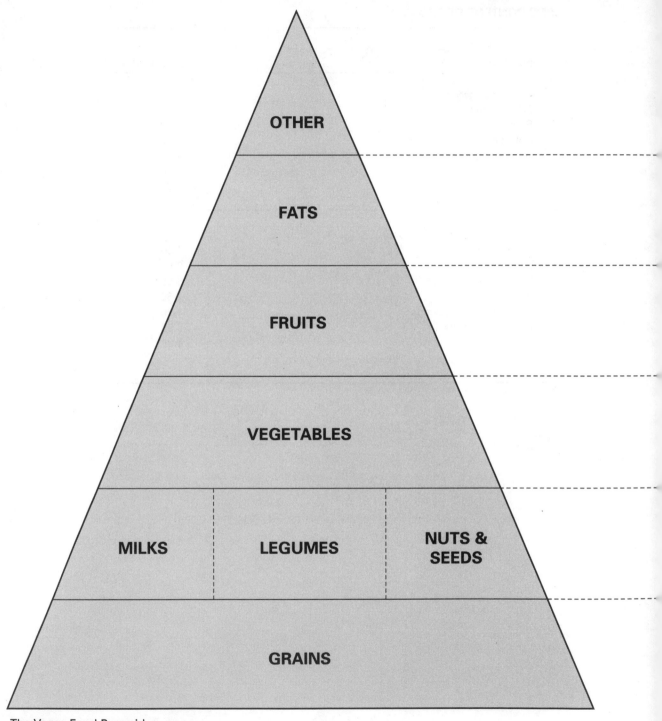

The Vegan Food Pyramid

Note: Amounts listed are a minimum number of servings.

TODDLERS & PRESCHOOL	SCHOOL AGED CHILDREN	ADOLESCENTS	ADULTS	PREGNANT & LACTATING WOMEN	FOOD AND SERVING SIZES
Optional	Optional	Optional	Optional	Optional	Soy cheese, baked sweets, snack chips. Serving sizes: 1 oz. cheese, 1 oz. snack chips, 2 oz. cookies or baked goods
3–4	5	4–6	2–3	2–3	Vegetable oil, margarine, salad dressing. Serving sizes: 1 teaspoon oil or margarine, 2 teaspoons salad dressing, 1 tablespoon low-fat salad dressing.
1–3	3	4	3	4	Apples, apricots, bananas, berries, cantaloupe, dates, figs, grapefruit, grapes, honeydew, kiwi, oranges, papaya, peaches, pears, persimmons, pineapple, plums, prunes, raisins, strawberries, watermelon, all fruit juices. Serving sizes: 1 piece fresh fruit, 1 wedge melon, ½ cup cooked or canned fruit, ¾ cup fruit juice, ¼ cup dried fruit.
1–2	4	4	4	5	Asparagus, beets, bok choy, broccoli, Brussels sprouts, cabbage, carrots, cauliflower, chard, collards, corn, eggplant, greens, jicama, kale, leeks, lettuce, mushrooms, okra, peas, peppers, potatoes, rutabagas, sea vegetables (dulse, kelp, nori, wakame), spinach, squash, sweet potatoes, tomatoes. Serving sizes: ½ cup cooked or 1 cup raw vegetables.
3–5*	4–5	6	5	6	Fortified soy or rice milk, black beans, black-eyed peas, chickpeas, great northern beans, kidney beans, lentils, limas, navy beans, pintos, soybeans, split peas, vegetarian baked beans, tempeh, textured vegetable protein, tofu, meat analogs, almonds, cashews, Brazil nuts, pecans, pine nuts, pistachios, walnuts, coconut, almond butter, peanut butter, tahini, pumpkin seeds, sesame seeds, sunflower seeds. Serving sizes: 1 cup milk, ½ cup cooked beans, tempeh, tofu, textured vegetable protein, 3 oz. meat analogs, 2 tablespoons nuts, nut butter, seeds.
3–4	6	10	8	7–8	Bread, cereal, cooked pasta, cooked rice or other grains, tortillas, pancakes, muffins, bagels, popcorn. Serving sizes: 1 slice bread, ½ cup cooked cereal, pasta, or grain, 8-inch tortilla, 1 pancake, 1 small muffin, ½ bagel, 2 cups popcorn.

* Include 1 serving of nuts or seeds and 3 cups of fortified soymilk daily.

MENU PLANNING USING THE VEGAN FOOD PYRAMID

Planning healthy vegan menus is easier than people might think. Concentrating on these five guidelines—which are based on the vegan food pyramid—will ensure taste, variety, and wholesomeness.

- Base menus on whole grains, vegetables, and fruits.
- Round meals out with moderate amounts of protein-rich foods, like beans, soy foods, and nondairy milks.
- Include moderate amounts of nuts, seeds, and nut or seed butters.
- Be sparing with added fats, and choose the healthiest ones, like olive and canola oil.
- Give attention to including plenty of calcium-rich foods in meals.

As you develop new menus that meet your needs, don't be too concerned about balanced meals. A balanced diet is one that includes a wide variety of plant foods, meets nutritional requirements, and has a calorie intake that is neither too high nor too low. But it isn't essential to strive for variety or complexity at every meal. A baked potato and a big bowl of steamed broccoli is a simple yet healthful vegan dinner. A bowl of cereal with fortified soymilk and fruit, or peanut butter and sliced banana on whole-wheat bread, is another quick and easy option. Individual meals don't have to be any more involved than this as long as you include a good variety of foods throughout the day. New vegans may feel slightly overwhelmed at the thought of coming up with a whole series of menus. Although many people believe they should eat something different for dinner every night of the month, the truth is that most eat and enjoy the same dozen or so meals over and over again. While some people are eager to experiment with new recipes, most will be content to rely on dishes they already know how to prepare and on convenience products that make meal planning a snap. Even the most novice cook can toss together a supper of baked potatoes, frozen veggie burgers, and steamed vegetables—or pasta with spaghetti sauce from a jar along with a tossed salad.

The menus that follow are ideas to get you started. Serving sizes are used to illustrate the guidelines in the vegan food pyramid. But you can estimate amounts and can also adjust the serving sizes to meet your calorie needs. The menus make liberal use of the recipes in this book to provide you with a comprehensive guide to vegan meal planning and cooking and to introduce you to some recipe ideas. If you don't have the time or desire to try new recipes right now, however, make the necessary adjustments to better suit your needs. For example, instead of following the recipe for orange-apricot oatmeal, you can make plain or instant oatmeal. Buy prepared hummus and canned or instant soups instead of making your own. Do keep your pantry and freezer stocked with some convenience items—frozen vegetables, instant soups, veggie burgers, canned beans, prepared spaghetti sauce, and ready-to-eat cereals. Having these foods on hand will make it easier for you to stick to a healthy vegan diet.

When using these menus or developing new ones, make it a point to select the most nutritious version of a food. For example, when a recipe calls for tofu, use the calcium-set variety. Choose calcium-fortified orange juice and fortified brands of soy and rice milk.

Nutritious snacks can round out and balance the diet. Each of the menus for adults and teens offers a list of snacks for that day, allowing you to choose when you will eat them. The menus for children specify three snacks per day, since frequent meals help small children meet calorie needs.

Recipes marked with an asterisk (*) are listed in Appendix C.

DAY ONE

Breakfast

Orange-apricot oatmeal*

2 slices whole-wheat toast

6 ounces apple juice

1 cup fortified rice milk

Lunch

Hummus sandwich with chopped tomatoes and lettuce* (½ cup hummus in whole-wheat pita pocket)

Carrot sticks

Apple

Dinner

Shells stuffed with tofu ricotta cheese* (1 cup shells, ½ cup tofu ricotta cheese)

Tossed salad with sunflower seed dressing*

Garlic bread

1 cup steamed kale

Snacks

¼ cup almonds

Fruit smoothie*

DAY TWO

Breakfast

Cereal with soymilk and sliced bananas

6 ounces orange juice

2 slices whole-wheat toast with margarine

Lunch

Pickle, tahini, and tomato sandwich*

Tossed salad with oil-and-vinegar dressing

2 fresh apricots

Ultimate chocolate-chip cookie*

Dinner

1 cup navy-bean soup*

2 slices seven-grain bread

1½ cups steamed broccoli and cauliflower

Snacks

Apple slices spread with 2 tablespoons peanut butter

DAY THREE

Breakfast

2 lemon-poppy-seed muffins*

6 ounces orange juice

1 cup hot spiced milk*

Lunch

1 cup navy-bean soup*

Salad with sunflower-seed dressing*

1 slice whole-wheat bread

2 fresh figs

Dinner

2 bean burritos*

1 cup brown rice

1 cup steamed kale

Ultimate chocolate-chip cookie*

Snacks

Apple slices spread with 2 table-spoons almond butter

DAY FOUR

Breakfast

Wheat-bran cereal with soymilk

6 ounces grapefruit juice

2 slices whole-wheat toast with fruit spread or margarine

Lunch

1 cup instant lentil soup

1 slice whole-wheat bread

2 kiwifruit

Dinner

1 cup spaghetti with prepared spaghetti sauce

Whole-grain Italian bread rubbed with garlic and drizzled with olive oil

Tossed salad with sunflower-seed dressing*

1 cup steamed or braised collards

½ cup canned apricots

Snacks

1 lemon-poppy-seed muffin*

1 cup almond milk

DAY FIVE

Breakfast

English muffin spread with 2 table-spoons soy-nut butter

Fruit smoothie*

Lunch

Curried tofu salad sandwich*

Carrot and celery sticks

Pear

Dinner

Veggie burger on a whole-wheat roll with ketchup, tomato slices, and pickles

Baked potato

1 cup steamed or braised collards

½ cup steamed carrots

Snacks

Bran muffin

1 cup soymilk

DAY SIX

Breakfast

2 slices French toast* with fruit-and-maple blend*

6 ounces orange juice

Lunch

½ cup tofu-vegetable spread* on 2 slices whole-grain toast

Salad with French dressing

Keepsake brownie*

Dinner

Saucy beans and franks*

½ cup hash-brown potatoes *(homemade or frozen; check packages, as some contain lard)*

1 cup steamed kale

1 cup steamed carrots

2 whole-wheat rolls

Snacks

Orange-banana whirl*

Bagel with fruit spread

DAY SEVEN

Breakfast

Shredded wheat with vanilla-flavored soymilk and blueberries

6 ounces orange juice

1 slice cinnamon-raisin toast spread with margarine

Lunch

1 cup instant black-bean soup

2 slices whole-wheat bread

Salad with oil-and-vinegar dressing

Carrot sticks

Dinner

Baked potatoes Florentine*

2 whole-wheat biscuits*

1 cup turnip greens

Fresh pineapple

Snacks

Keepsake brownie*

1 cup soymilk

Banana

SAMPLE MENU FOR TODDLERS

(Adjust serving sizes for your toddler, since appetites vary among children and in the same child from day to day.)

Breakfast

¼ cup cinnamon-apple oatmeal*

½ cup orange juice

Snack

1 graham cracker

1 cup vanilla soymilk

Lunch

½ peanut-butter-and-banana sandwich on whole-wheat bread

¼ cup carrot-and-raisin salad with vegan mayonnaise

Snack

½ cup fruit smoothie*

Dinner

¼ cup mashed potatoes

¼ cup vegetarian baked beans

¼ cup steamed green beans

Snack:

½ slice bread spread with 1 tablespoon almond butter

SAMPLE MENU FOR PRESCHOOLERS

(Adjust serving sizes for your preschooler since appetites vary among children and in the same child from day to day.)

Breakfast

1 slice French toast* with fruit-and-maple blend*

½ cup orange juice

Snack

½ bagel with fruit spread

Lunch

½ hummus sandwich*

Carrot sticks

½ cup canned pears

1 cup soymilk

Snack

Crackers spread with 1 tablespoon almond butter

Dinner

Shells stuffed with tofu ricotta cheese*

½ cup steamed peas

1 slice whole-grain bread

Sliced banana

Snack

½ cup vegetable soup

SAMPLE MENU FOR TEENS

MENU ONE

Breakfast

Fruit smoothie*

Bagel spread with 2 tablespoons peanut butter

Lunch

2 pitas stuffed with ½ cup monster mash spread*

Carrot sticks

Banana

2 oatmeal cookies

Orange juice

Dinner *(with friends)*

3 slices cheeseless pizza topped with vegetables

Salad with French dressing

Soft drink or juice

Snacks

¼ cup trail mix

Bran flakes with 1 cup soymilk

Apple slices spread with 2 tablespoons almond butter

SAMPLE MENU FOR TEENS

MENU TWO

Breakfast

Bran flakes with 1 cup soymilk

2 slices whole-wheat toast with fruit spread

Banana

Lunch

Tempeh burger on whole-wheat roll with sliced tomato and lettuce

Peach

6 ounces orange juice

Keepsake brownie*

Dinner

1½ cups vegetarian chili made from mix

1 cup brown rice

1 cup steamed broccoli

1 cup steamed carrots

1 slice whole-grain bread

Snacks

Shredded wheat with sliced banana and 1 cup soymilk

1 lemon-poppy-seed muffin*

English muffin with almond butter spread

Apple

1 cup rice milk

SPECIAL INGREDIENTS AND VEGAN RECIPES

SPECIAL INGREDIENTS

Balsamic vinegar is an exquisitely flavored seasoning made from white Trebbiano grape juice that acquires a dark amber color and pungent sweetness after aging for three to thirty years in barrels made from various woods—red oak, chestnut, mulberry, and juniper. The finest balsamics are slightly sweet, heavy, mellow, and dark.

Brown rice vinegar is a mild vinegar made from fermented rice. It is widely used in Japanese and Chinese cooking and adds a light Asian flavor to sauces and dressings. Traditionally, the vinegar is brewed in earthenware crocks. It is then filtered and aged in casks until the flavor is mellow and the color is deep amber.

Bulgur is hard red winter wheat that has been cracked and toasted. It comes in coarse, medium, and fine grinds. Bulgur cooks quickly. It has a chewy, "meaty" texture and a delicious nutty flavor.

Flaxseeds are rich in fiber and omega-3 fatty acids and make an excellent substitute for eggs in baking. To use them for this purpose, finely grind 1 tablespoon flaxseeds in an electric herb or coffee mill or in a dry blender. Place in a blender along with 3 tablespoons water and process until frothy and viscous. This will make the equivalent of one medium egg for use in baking. If time permits, let the mixture rest in the refrigerator for an hour or more before using. It can also be stored in the refrigerator for up to three days. Flaxseeds are available in natural food stores. They are highly perishable and should be stored in the freezer to prevent rancidity.

Millet is an ancient grain native to the East Indies and North Africa. It has a tiny round yellowish seed (resembling a mustard seed) and a mild, slightly nutty flavor. Millet is gluten-free, easily digestible, and one of the least allergenic foods known. It contains abundant minerals, vitamins, protein, and fiber. When cooked, millet swells to a fluffy texture. Toasting it before cooking enhances the flavor and creates a more pilaflike result. With extra water, it can be cooked into a tasty breakfast porridge. Available in natural-food stores. Store at room temperature or in the freezer.

Miso is a salty, flavorful, fermented bean paste that often contains rice, barley, or another grain. Used primarily as a seasoning, miso ranges from dark and strongly flavored to light, smooth, and delicately flavored. Light misos are generally sweeter and less salty than dark misos. Look for unpasteurized (refrigerated) varieties in natural-food stores.

Naturally brewed soy sauce (tamari and shoyu) is produced by the natural fermentation of soybeans, salt, water, and sometimes wheat. (Naturally brewed soy sauce is called *shoyu* if wheat is used, *tamari* if it is not.) The finest soy sauces are aged for a year or longer. With time, you will develop as discriminating a taste for tamari and shoyu as some people have for fine wine. Store tamari or shoyu at room temperature or in the refrigerator for optimum flavor. It will keep indefinitely. For a lower sodium content, look for reduced-sodium or "lite" tamari.

Nutritional yeast is a natural whole plant grown as a food crop. It is prized for its delicious, nutty taste and high nutritional content. When mixed with certain seasonings, nutritional yeast can also impart a cheesy taste or a poultrylike flavor. Red Star brand Vegetarian Support Formula (VSF) nutritional yeast is a concentrated source of protein and a good source of B-complex vitamins, including vitamin B_{12}. It contains no fat and has few calories. The B_{12} in Red Star VSF nutritional yeast is from natural fermentation and is not obtained from a synthetic process or derived from an animal source. This is an easy, delicious, and reliable way to incorporate vitamin B_{12} into the vegan diet.

If you are unable to locate Red Star Vegetarian Support Formula nutritional yeast in your area, it may be ordered from The Mail Order Catalog, Box 180, Summertown, Tennessee 38483. For current price information, call 1-800-695-2241.

Organic flaxseed oil is an abundant source of omega-3 fatty acids, one of the essential fatty acids most often lacking in modern diets. Omega-3 fatty acids have been credited with amazing healing and preventive properties. Using flaxseed oil as a salad dressing and drizzling it over cooked foods (such as a baked potato) are the easiest and most nutritious ways to incorporate it into your daily diet.

Because flaxseed oil is prone to rancidity and highly susceptible to nutrient loss from exposure to air, light, and heat, special care must be taken when purchasing and storing it and when using it in recipes. Always keep flaxseed oil in the refrigerator. Recap it immediately after use and return it to the refrigerator as soon as possible. Never heat flaxseed oil or use it in cooking. Purchase only refrigerated flaxseed oil in small quantities (no more than 10 to 12 ounces at a time). It should come packaged in a light-impervious plastic or dark glass bottle that is stamped with a freshness date. Use it up within two to three weeks after opening the bottle.

Quinoa is a quick-cooking, gluten-free grain native to the Andes. Its small, disk-shaped seeds look like a cross between sesame seeds and millet. It has more calcium than cow's milk, is high in protein, rich in minerals, and easy to digest. Rinse well under cold running water before cooking to remove its bitter coating. Store in the freezer.

Regular tofu is water-packed tofu typically found in plastic tubs in the refrigerated section of your natural-food store and in the produce section of some supermarkets. Look for tofu processed with calcium salts for the highest calcium content.

Salsa is a condiment or dip featuring tomatoes, chilies, and cilantro. Store opened jars in the refrigerator.

Seitan, also called wheat meat, is a high-protein, fat-free food made from the protein (i.e., gluten) in wheat. It has a meaty texture and flavor and makes an ideal meat substitute in many traditional recipes. It is available in the deli case or freezer of natural-food stores.

Silken tofu is a smooth, creamy, delicate tofu that is excellent for blending into sauces, dips, cream soups, and puddings. It is often available in special aseptic packaging that allows storage without refrigeration for up to a year (you'll need to refrigerate it after opening). One popular brand, Mori-Nu, is available in most grocery stores. Other brands of silken tofu can be found in the refrigerated section of supermarkets and natural-food stores.

Tahini is a paste made by grinding raw or lightly toasted whole or hulled sesame seeds. It is light tan in color and rich and creamy like peanut butter. The consistency of tahini varies from brand to brand; some types are creamy and smooth, and others are oily or dry. Seek out tahini made from organically grown sesame seeds for the best flavor and quality. Pour off the excess oil that rises to the top. Stir well and store in the refrigerator in an airtight container.

ORANGE-APRICOT OATMEAL

Serves 2

A chewy and satisfying hot cereal with just a hint of sweetness. Dried apricots are an excellent source of vitamin A, iron, and potassium. Seek out only organic dried apricots. They will be a deep orange-brown color. Avoid ones that are bright orange, as they will have been treated with sulfur dioxide.

1. Place all the ingredients except the maple syrup, flaxseed oil, and nuts in a medium saucepan and stir to combine. Bring to a boil. Cover and reduce heat to low. Simmer for 5 minutes, stirring once or twice.
2. Remove from heat and let sit, covered, for 2 to 5 minutes.
3. Stir in maple syrup and flaxseed oil, if using. Sprinkle one tablespoon nuts over each serving, if desired.

TIP:
To pan-toast the nuts, lightly dry-roast them in a skillet over medium heat, stirring often, until fragrant and golden brown.

1 cup old-fashioned rolled oats

1¼ cups cold water

½ cup orange juice (or 2 tablespoons frozen orange-juice concentrate plus 6 tablespoons water)

2 tablespoons finely chopped dried apricots

¼ teaspoon ground nutmeg

Tiny pinch of salt

2 tablespoons pure maple syrup (optional)

2 teaspoons organic flaxseed oil (optional)

2 tablespoons chopped walnuts, pecans, or almonds, lightly pan-toasted if desired (optional)

CINNAMON-APPLE OATMEAL

Serves 2

Old-fashioned rolled oats make a hearty morning meal. If you prefer, use dates or raisins instead of or in addition to the dried apples.

1	cup old-fashioned rolled oats
1¼	cups cold water
½	cup apple juice (or 2 tablespoons frozen juice concentrate plus 6 tablespoons water)
2	tablespoons finely chopped dried apples
¼	teaspoon ground cinnamon
	Tiny pinch of salt
2	tablespoons pure maple syrup (optional)
2	teaspoons organic flaxseed oil (optional)
2	tablespoons chopped walnuts, pecans, or almonds, lightly pan-toasted if desired (optional)

1. Place all the ingredients except the maple syrup, flaxseed oil, and nuts in a medium saucepan and stir to combine. Bring to a boil. Cover and reduce heat to low. Simmer for 5 minutes, stirring once or twice.
2. Remove from heat and let sit, covered, for 2 to 5 minutes.
3. Stir in maple syrup and flaxseed oil, if using. Sprinkle one tablespoon nuts over each serving, if desired.

TIP:

To pan-toast the nuts, lightly dry-roast them in a skillet over medium heat, stirring often, until fragrant and golden brown.

LEMON–POPPY-SEED MUFFINS

Fragrant, zesty, crunchy, and moist, these delectable muffins will arouse all your senses.

1. Preheat the oven to 375 degrees F. Lightly oil the bottoms and sides of 12 muffin cups with canola oil or nonstick cooking spray.
2. Place the flour, poppy seeds, baking powder, baking soda, and salt in a large mixing bowl and stir them with a wire whisk until well combined.
3. Place the flaxseeds in a dry blender and grind them into a powder. Add ½ cup of the water and blend until a gummy mixture is achieved, about 30 seconds. Add the remaining ½ cup of water, apple-juice concentrate, lemon juice, oil, maple syrup, lemon zest, and vanilla and process until frothy and well blended, between 1 and 2 minutes. Pour into the flour mixture and mix just until everything is evenly moistened. The batter will be stiff.
4. Quickly spoon the batter into the prepared muffin cups, filling each cup almost to the top. Bake immediately on the center shelf of the oven until a toothpick inserted in the center of a muffin comes out clean, about 18 to 20 minutes.
5. Cool the muffins in the pan on a rack for 2 minutes. Run a knife around the edge of each muffin, then carefully loosen the muffins and turn them out onto a cooling rack. Serve warm or cool completely before storing in an airtight container in the refrigerator for future use.

2	cups whole-wheat pastry flour
½	cup barley flour (or additional whole-wheat pastry flour)
¼	cup poppy seeds
2	teaspoons double-acting nonaluminum baking powder
1	teaspoon baking soda
¼	teaspoon salt
2	tablespoons flaxseeds
1	cup water
½	cup frozen apple-juice concentrate, thawed
⅓	cup fresh lemon juice (remove the zest from the lemons before juicing)
⅓	cup canola oil
⅓	cup pure maple syrup
2	tablespoons lemon zest (colored part only; organic if possible)
1	teaspoon vanilla extract

SPICED DATE AND NUT SCONES

Makes 12 scones

Walnuts and dates make an appealing combination in these light and tender pastries.

1. Preheat the oven to 375 degrees F. Lightly oil a baking sheet or mist it with nonstick cooking spray, and set it aside.

2. Place the flour, rolled oats, baking powder, cinnamon, baking soda, allspice, cardamom, and salt in a large mixing bowl and stir them with a wire whisk until well combined. Stir in the dates and walnuts, making sure that the date pieces are coated with flour and do not stick together.

3. Place the flaxseeds in a dry blender and grind them into a powder. Add the water and blend until a gummy mixture is achieved, about 30 seconds. Add the milk, oil, maple syrup, and vanilla and process until frothy and well blended, about 1 to 2 minutes. Pour into the flour mixture and mix just until everything is evenly moistened.

4. Using a ⅓ cup measure per scone, drop the batter in dollops onto the prepared baking sheet, leaving about 2 inches between dollops. (You may need to scoop out the batter from the

2	cups whole-wheat pastry flour
1	cup old-fashioned rolled oats
2	teaspoons double-acting nonaluminum baking powder
1	teaspoon ground cinnamon
1	teaspoon baking soda
¼	teaspoon allspice
¼	teaspoon cardamom
¼	teaspoon salt
1	cup chopped pitted dates, packed
½	cup chopped walnuts
2	tablespoons flaxseeds
½	cup water
½	cup plain nondairy milk (or water)
⅓	cup canola oil
⅓	cup pure maple syrup
1	teaspoon vanilla extract
2	tablespoons sugar
½	teaspoon ground cinnamon

measuring cup with a spoon, rubber spatula, or your fingers.) Flatten the scones slightly into irregular shapes about 3 inches in diameter.

5. Combine the sugar with the cinnamon in a small bowl. Sprinkle the mixture generously over the top of the scones.

6. Bake on the center shelf of the oven for 12 to14 minutes, or until golden brown. With a spatula, transfer the scones to a cooling rack. Serve hot or warm. Cool leftovers completely before storing in an airtight container in the refrigerator for future use.

WHOLE-WHEAT BISCUITS

Makes about 10 biscuits

Serve these wholesome, flaky biscuits warm with applesauce or fruit-sweetened jam.

- 2 cups whole-wheat pastry flour
- 1 tablespoon double-acting nonaluminum baking powder
- ½ teaspoon salt
- ⅓ cup canola oil

  Approximately ½ cup plain nondairy milk, more or less as needed

1. Preheat the oven to 450 degrees F. Whisk together the flour, baking powder, and salt in a large mixing bowl. Cut in the oil with a fork or pastry blender until the mixture resembles coarse crumbs.
2. Using a fork, stir in just enough of the milk so that the dry ingredients are moistened and the dough comes together. (Too much milk will make the dough sticky; too little will make the biscuits dry.)
3. Gather the dough in a ball and turn it out onto a lightly floured work surface. Knead it gently 20 to 25 times. Then smooth it into a ball. Roll or pat the dough into a ½-inch thick round and cut it with a floured 2½-inch biscuit cutter or the rim of a glass. Push the cutter straight down into the dough without twisting it. Reroll and recut the scraps of dough. Place the biscuits on an ungreased baking sheet about an inch apart for crusty sides or touching for soft sides.
4. Bake on the center shelf of the oven for 10 to 12 minutes, or until the bottoms are lightly browned. Do not overbake. Serve hot or warm.

VARIATIONS

For Cornmeal Biscuits:
Substitute ½ cup yellow cornmeal for ½ cup flour. Sprinkle a little cornmeal over the biscuits before baking them, if desired.

For Drop Biscuits:
Increase the milk to approximately ¾ cup, using just enough to make a very thick batter. Instead of using a fork, stir the batter with a wooden spoon. Mist the baking sheet with nonstick cooking spray and drop the dough by large rounded spoonfuls onto it to make 10 biscuits.

FLAXJACKS

Makes about a dozen 3-inch pancakes (Serves 3 to 4)

These tender pancakes are great for leisurely mornings when you don't need to rush. They are light, fluffy, and fabulous.

1 cup whole-wheat pastry flour

2 teaspoons double-acting nonaluminum baking powder

⅛ teaspoon salt

1 tablespoon flaxseeds

¼ cup water

¾ cup plain nondairy milk

1 tablespoon canola oil, plus extra as needed for cooking

1 tablespoon sugar

½ teaspoon vanilla extract

1. Place the flour, baking powder, and salt in a medium mixing bowl and stir them together.

2. Place the flaxseeds in a dry blender and grind them into a powder. Add the water and blend until a gummy mixture is achieved, about 30 seconds. Add the milk, oil, sugar, and vanilla extract and process until frothy and well blended, about 1 to 2 minutes. Pour into the flour mixture and mix just until everything is evenly moistened.

3. Coat a skillet or griddle with a little canola oil, and heat it over medium-high. Spoon the batter into the hot skillet using about 2 tablespoons for each pancake.

4. Cook until bubbles pop through the top of the pancakes and the bottoms are golden brown, about 2 to 3 minutes. Turn the pancakes over and cook until they are golden and cooked through, about 1 minute longer.

TIP:

Be sure to add a little canola oil to the skillet between each batch to prevent the pancakes from sticking to the pan. To keep the finished pancakes warm while the remainder cook, place them on a baking sheet in a 300-degree F. oven. This way you can serve the pancakes hot all at the same time and no one has to wait.

FRENCH TOAST

Serves 2 to 3

Serve warm with buttery-tasting Flaxen Maple Syrup, p. 268.

¼ cup whole-wheat pastry flour

1 teaspoon nutritional yeast flakes (optional)

¼ teaspoon salt

Pinch *each* ground cinnamon and nutmeg

1 cup nondairy milk (plain or vanilla)

6 slices whole-grain bread

1. Place the dry ingredients in a medium mixing bowl and whisk until well blended. Pour the milk into the flour and whisk vigorously until well blended. Let the batter sit for 10 minutes.

2. Oil a skillet or griddle and heat it over medium-high. Mix the batter again. Dip the bread slices, one at a time, into the batter, making sure that both sides are well saturated. Cook 3 to 5 minutes until the bottom is lightly browned, then turn over and cook the other side until browned.

TIP:

This French toast tends to stick to the pan during cooking. Use a nonstick pan for the best results, or be sure to oil the pan well between batches.

FRUIT-AND-MAPLE BLEND

Makes about ½ cup

This luscious mixture is an ideal topping for pancakes, French toast, or hot cereal.

¼ cup pure maple syrup

¼ cup berries (or peeled and finely chopped fresh fruit)

Combine the maple syrup and fruit in a small bowl or measuring cup and stir well. For a smoother consistency, combine the mixture in a blender and process until lightly blended.

TIP:

Fruit-sweetened preserves may be substituted for the fresh fruit, if preferred. If the preserves are very thick, stir them well, then thin with a little water, if necessary, before combining with the maple syrup. This recipe is easily doubled, tripled, or quadrupled. It's great when you're cooking for a crowd and want an easy, delicious topping that tastes really special but doesn't require much work.

FLAXEN MAPLE SYRUP

Makes about ½ cup

Flaxseed oil adds luscious buttery taste and essential omega-3 fatty acids to this sweetly simple recipe.

½ cup pure maple syrup

2 teaspoons organic flaxseed oil

Place the maple syrup in a small mixing bowl. Add the flaxseed oil and whisk until well blended.

HOT SPICED MILK

Serves 1

This soothing beverage is based on a recipe from my friend Sonal Sheth, who made it for me when I visited her and her family in California. It is fragrant, warming, and delightful. Sonal suggests you make it with half rice milk and half soymilk for a rich but not-too-sweet taste.

1 cup plain nondairy milk
¼ teaspoon ground cardamom
⅛ teaspoon ground cinnamon
Pinch of ground black pepper
Large pinch of saffron threads
Sugar, as desired

1. Combine the milk, cardamom, cinnamon, pepper, and saffron in a small saucepan and whisk them together. Place over medium heat, stirring occasionally until hot.
2. Pour the milk through a fine strainer to filter out the spices (you can put the strainer over your cup or mug and pour the hot milk directly into it). Stir in as much sugar as necessary to achieve the desired sweetness. Serve hot.

TIP:
This recipe is easily doubled, tripled, or quadrupled. It's a tasty hot beverage for mornings or evenings and makes a satisfying replacement for caffeinated drinks. It's also suitable for children (just go easy on the black pepper which may be too spicy for younger tastes).

HOT COCOA

Serves 2

Hot cocoa made with plant milk (soy, rice, nut, or grain) is rich, smooth, and satisfying. Everyone knows hot cocoa is wonderful in cool weather, but this recipe is so simple and delicious it may become a year-round favorite.

3 tablespoons unsweetened cocoa powder

3 tablespoons sugar

½ cup water

2 cups nondairy milk

½ teaspoon vanilla extract

1. Combine the cocoa, sugar, and water in a small saucepan, and whisk until smooth. Place over medium heat, stirring constantly, until the mixture comes to a boil. Simmer, stirring constantly, for 1 minute.

2. Whisk in the milk and cook, stirring often, until steam rises and the mixture is hot. Do not boil. Stir in the vanilla. Pour into mugs and serve at once.

TIP:
This recipe is easily doubled, tripled, or quadrupled.

FRUIT SMOOTHIE

Serves 2

A creamy, refreshing shake without any dairy products.

Cut the banana into chunks and place it along with the remaining ingredients in a blender. Process until smooth and creamy. Serve at once.

1	medium banana, frozen
1½	cups fruit juice of your choice
½	cup peeled and sliced fresh fruit or berries

ORANGE-BANANA WHIRL

Serves 2

This nutritious shake makes a refreshing snack.

Cut the banana into chunks. Place all ingredients in a blender and process until smooth and creamy. Serve at once.

TIP:
To freeze a banana, peel it and wrap it tightly in plastic wrap or place it in an airtight storage container. Put it in the freezer for several hours or overnight, until it is solidly frozen.

1	small banana, frozen
1⅔	cups orange juice (or ¼ cup orange-juice concentrate plus ¾ cup ice water)
¼ to ½	teaspoon vanilla extract, to taste

271

ALMOND-FLAX BUTTER

Makes about ½ cup

Use this golden spread, rich in omega-3 fatty acids, as a replacement for dairy butter on toasted bread, bagels, or crackers.

½ cup raw almonds

3 tablespoons organic flaxseed oil

Pinch of salt, to taste

1. If your almonds have skins, they will need to be blanched and peeled: Place them in a small saucepan and cover them with water; bring to a boil, reduce the heat slightly, and simmer for 2 minutes. Drain the almonds in a colander and rinse them under cold water. Pop off the skins by pinching the base of each almond between your thumb and forefinger. Pat the almonds dry. (These first steps are unnecessary if you are using skinless almonds.)

2. Grind the almonds into a meal in a food processor fitted with a metal blade. Add the oil one tablespoon at a time, and process until creamy. Add salt to taste. Store in an airtight container in the refrigerator.

HUMMUS

The best of the beloved bean dips.

1. Place the beans in a food processor fitted with a metal blade and process until they are ground.
2. Add the tahini, lemon juice, and oil and process into a coarse paste, adding about a tablespoon of water only if necessary to facilitate processing.
3. Add the remaining ingredients and blend thoroughly.

1⅔ cups soft-cooked garbanzo beans, rinsed and drained

¼ cup tahini

3 tablespoons fresh lemon juice

1 tablespoon organic flaxseed oil or extra-virgin olive oil

1 tablespoon water, more or less if needed

2 tablespoons chopped fresh parsley

½ teaspoon minced garlic

¼ teaspoon ground cumin

¼ teaspoon ground coriander

¼ teaspoon paprika

Pinch of salt (or to taste)

Pinch of cayenne pepper

MONSTER MASH

Makes about 1 cup

This is a fun, creative spread that calls for a little ingenuity. Start with your choice of beans and add one or more ingredients to suit your taste, making the spread as thick or thin as you like. Kids especially enjoy inventing their own Monster Mash recipes. Use the finished "mash" as a sandwich filling, a spread for crackers, or dip for chips and veggies.

1. Place the beans in a food processor fitted with a metal blade and process until they are ground.
2. Add the optional ingredients of your choice and process into a coarse paste, adding bean liquid or water, as needed. Taste; then adjust seasonings and add more optional ingredients as necessary to achieve the flavor and texture you desire.

1 cup soft-cooked beans of your choice, drained (reserve liquid)

OPTIONAL INGREDIENTS

Barbecue sauce

Capers

Carrot (minced or shredded)

Citrus juice (lemon, lime, or orange)

Garlic

Herbs (fresh or dried)

Horseradish

Ketchup

Lemon juice

Mustard

Nut or seed butter

Nutritional yeast flakes

Oil (extra-virgin olive or organic flaxseed)

Onion (Vidalia or red; scallions; shallots)

Pickles (chopped or relish)

Salt and pepper

Spices

Tamari

Tomato paste

Mayonnaise (egg- and dairy-free)

Salad dressing (nondairy)

Vegetables, cooked

Vinegar

SOUR CREAM AND ONION DIP

Makes about 1 cup

An irresistible chip and vegetable dip that also makes a terrific topping for baked potatoes.

Place all the ingredients in a food processor and process until well combined. Transfer to a covered container and store in the refrigerator. Let rest several hours before serving to allow flavors to blend.

1 cup silken tofu (firm)
2 tablespoons canola oil
1 tablespoon dried onion flakes
1 tablespoon fresh lemon juice
1 tablespoon apple cider vinegar
1 teaspoon tamari
1 teaspoon sugar
¼ teaspoon dried parsley flakes (optional)

SESAME-MISO SPREAD

Makes about ⅓ cup

This buttery-tasting spread is very rich. Spread it thinly on toast or crackers or use it as a replacement for peanut butter.

Combine the miso, tahini, flaxseed oil, and sesame oil in a small bowl and stir them into a smooth paste. Vigorously stir in the water, using enough to make the mixture spreadable (it should be similar in consistency to peanut butter). Use at once or store in an airtight container in the refrigerator.

2 tablespoons sweet white miso
2 tablespoons tahini
1 teaspoon organic flaxseed oil
1 teaspoon dark sesame oil
2 tablespoons water, as needed

SPICY PEANUT DIP

Makes about 1¼ cups

This versatile mixture can be used as a sauce for steamed vegetables, pasta, grains, or potatoes. It's also a great dip for crisp carrot and zucchini sticks, bell pepper strips, cauliflower and broccoli flowerets, and toasted pita wedges.

Place all the ingredients in a food processor fitted with a metal blade and process until well blended. Alternatively, mash all the ingredients together in a medium-size mixing bowl. Taste; then add more lemon juice or Tabasco sauce, if desired.

½ cup peanut butter

½ cup prepared salsa

3 tablespoons fresh lemon juice

1 teaspoon sugar

½ teaspoon ground cumin

Several drops Tabasco sauce, to taste

Pinch of salt, to taste

TOFU-VEGETABLE SPREAD

Makes about 1½ cups

This quick and easy pâté is so impressively delicious that no one will guess it took mere minutes to make.

½ pound firm regular tofu

2 tablespoons tahini

1 tablespoon sweet white miso

2 teaspoons tamari (or to taste)

½ cup shredded carrot

¼ cup sliced scallions

1. Steam or simmer the tofu in water for 10 minutes. Cool.
2. Crumble the tofu and place it in a food processor fitted with a metal blade. Add the tahini, miso, and tamari and process into a thick paste. Add the carrot and scallions and pulse until they are evenly distributed. Transfer to a storage container and chill several hours before serving.

WILTED SPINACH SALAD WITH RASPBERRY VINAIGRETTE

Serves 4

This scrumptious salad is effortless to prepare, making it perfect for everyday service, but its elegant presentation also makes it ideal for company.

1. Remove the stems of the spinach, and rinse the leaves well. Dry the leaves thoroughly by either patting them with a clean kitchen towel or spinning them in a salad spinner. Tear the spinach leaves into large pieces, and place them in a large mixing bowl along with the mushrooms and onion.

2. To make the dressing, heat the oil in a small skillet or saucepan. Add the garlic and stir-fry it for 30 seconds. Then add the raspberry jelly, vinegar, salt, and pepper. Warm the dressing just until the jelly is melted and bubbly. Remove the pan from the heat.

3. Pour the warm dressing over the spinach leaves, mushrooms, and onion. Toss until everything is evenly coated. Top each serving with a tablespoon of the seeds or nuts. Serve at once.

TIP:
To pan-toast the sunflower seeds or walnuts, lightly dry-roast them in a skillet over medium heat, stirring often, until fragrant and golden brown.

SALAD MIX

6 cups fresh spinach leaves (stems removed), torn and lightly packed

1 cup thinly sliced mushrooms

2 very thin slices red onion, cut in half and separated into crescents

RASPBERRY VINAIGRETTE

1½ tablespoons extra-virgin olive oil

1 teaspoon minced garlic

2 tablespoons fruit-sweetened seedless raspberry jelly

2 tablespoons red wine vinegar

⅛ teaspoon salt (or to taste)

Pinch of ground black pepper, to taste

¼ cup sunflower seeds or coarsely chopped walnuts, lightly pan-toasted (see tip)

UNRULY TABOULI

Serves 4 to 6

Although this Middle Eastern grain salad doesn't take much time or effort to prepare, it must marinate in the refrigerator for several hours to properly soften the bulgur. It's worth the wait, however, as the long marinating time ensures each grain is infused with eye-popping flavor.

1. Place the bulgur in a heatproof mixing bowl. Dissolve the salt in the boiling water and pour over the bulgur. Mix well, cover, and let sit for 30 minutes.
2. Combine the lemon juice, olive oil, and flaxseed oil and add to the bulgur.
3. Stir in the parsley, scallions, spearmint, and garlic and mix well. Cover tightly and marinate the salad in the refrigerator for 4 to 12 hours. Toss or top with your choice of optional additions shortly before serving.

TIP:

When options are added, this tabouli comes into its own and is transformed from an auxiliary dish to the main attraction. Just add a light soup and warm pita bread to round out the meal.

1 cup bulgur (fine or medium grind)

1½ cups boiling water

1 teaspoon salt

¼ cup fresh lemon juice

2 tablespoons extra-virgin olive oil

2 tablespoons organic flaxseed oil (or additional olive oil)

1 cup finely chopped parsley, firmly packed

4 scallions, thinly sliced (green and white parts)

1½ teaspoons dried spearmint

½ teaspoon minced garlic

UNRULY OPTIONS

1 cup soft-cooked or canned garbanzo beans

1 cup diced English cucumber

½ to 1 cup additional chopped parsley

1 ripe tomato, diced

½ cup sliced red radishes

½ cup finely minced bell pepper (red, yellow, or green)

½ cup grated carrot

279

TANG TSEL

Serves 4

Although this wonderful Tibetan-style coleslaw is made with just a few staple ingredients, it makes an amazingly delectable salad that even children love.

1 cup green cabbage, thinly sliced (or shredded)

1 cup red cabbage, thinly sliced (or shredded)

1 small ripe tomato, seeded and sliced into thin slivers

¼ cup brown rice vinegar

2 tablespoons dark sesame oil

1. Place the cabbage and tomato in a medium mixing bowl and toss them together.
2. Sprinkle the vinegar and sesame oil over the vegetables and toss again to mix thoroughly.

EASY ITALIAN DRESSING

Makes about ½ cup

Combine all ingredients in a mixing bowl and beat well with a wire whisk until emulsified.

3 tablespoons extra-virgin olive oil

3 tablespoons red wine vinegar

1 tablespoon organic flaxseed oil (or additional olive oil)

1 tablespoon fresh lemon juice

1 teaspoon Dijon mustard

1 teaspoon dried basil

½ teaspoon minced garlic

½ teaspoon sugar

¼ teaspoon dried oregano

¼ teaspoon dried thyme

¼ teaspoon salt (or to taste)

Ground black pepper (or cayenne pepper), to taste

SUNFLOWER-SEED DRESSING

Makes about 1 cup

A delightfully creamy and mild dressing.

Place the sunflower seeds in a blender and grind them into a powder. Add the remaining ingredients and process several minutes, until creamy and smooth.

½ cup hulled sunflower seeds

⅔ cup water

3 tablespoons extra-virgin olive oil

3 tablespoons fresh lemon juice

1 tablespoon organic flaxseed oil (or additional olive oil)

1 tablespoon tamari

1 teaspoon dried tarragon

1 teaspoon dried dill

½ teaspoon minced garlic

MISO MASTER DRESSING

Makes about ¾ cup

Combine all ingredients in a blender or food processor and process until smooth.

3 tablespoons sweet white miso

2 tablespoons extra-virgin olive oil

2 tablespoons organic flaxseed oil (or additional olive oil)

2 tablespoons water

2 tablespoons brown-rice vinegar

2 tablespoons brown-rice syrup

2 tablespoons chopped onion

1 teaspoon Dijon mustard

SWEET TOMATO VINAIGRETTE

Makes about 1 cup

Combine all ingredients in a blender or food processor and process until smooth and well blended.

¼ cup ketchup

¼ cup orange juice

¼ cup brown rice vinegar

3 tablespoons extra-virgin olive oil

2 tablespoons sugar

1 tablespoon organic flaxseed oil (or additional olive oil)

½ teaspoon minced garlic

¼ teaspoon salt

¼ teaspoon ground black pepper

POWER DRESSING

Makes about ⅓ cup

Combine all ingredients in a small bowl and whisk until well combined.

2 tablespoons nutritional yeast flakes

2 tablespoons extra-virgin olive oil

1 tablespoon organic flaxseed oil (or additional olive oil)

1 tablespoon fresh lemon juice

1 tablespoon water

½ teaspoon tamari

RED GAZPACHO

Makes 1 quart

A warm-weather delight, this "liquefied salad" is light and spicy.

1. Combine all the ingredients *except the optional garnishes* in a blender. Pulse the blender briefly, just until everything is well combined but the vegetables are still somewhat chunky.
2. Transfer the soup to a covered storage container, and chill it in the refrigerator for several hours before serving.
3. Serve the soup cold. Garnish each serving with a dollop of tofu sour cream, avocado chunks, and/or a few fresh cilantro leaves, if desired.

2 cups canned whole tomatoes, with juice, coarsely chopped

1½ cups chunked English cucumber

1 cup tomato juice

1 very small (or ½ of a large) yellow, red, or orange bell pepper, chopped

½ cup chopped red onion

3 tablespoons fresh lemon juice

3 tablespoons red-wine vinegar (or 1 to 2 tablespoons apple-cider vinegar)

1 tablespoon extra-virgin olive oil

½ teaspoon minced garlic

¼ teaspoon ground black pepper (or to taste)

Several drops Tabasco sauce (or to taste)

OPTIONAL GARNISHES

Tofu sour cream, (see p. 310)

Avocado chunks

Fresh cilantro leaves

BROCCOLI BISQUE AMANDINE

Makes about 5 cups

Sweet, creamy almonds are a lovely foil to the slightly bitter taste of broccoli. The enchanting flavor defies the simplicity of the ingredients.

⅓ cup blanched whole almonds, ground (see tip)

6 cups broccoli flowerets

2½ cups plain nondairy milk

Salt and ground black pepper to taste

1. Preheat the oven to 350 degrees F. Spread the ground almonds in a thin, even layer on a dry baking sheet, and toast them in the oven for 8 to 10 minutes, just until they are golden. (Watch closely so that the almonds do not burn!) Reserve 4 teaspoons of the toasted ground almonds for a garnish, and set the remainder aside.

2. Steam the broccoli until it is very tender, about 12 to 14 minutes. Combine the cooked broccoli, remaining toasted ground almonds, and the milk in batches in a blender. Process each batch until the mixture is completely smooth. Pour the blended soup into a large mixing bowl and continue processing the rest of the soup in a similar fashion.

3. Transfer the blended mixture to a 2-quart saucepan. Warm the soup over medium heat, stirring often until it is hot. Do not boil. Season the soup with salt and pepper to taste. Sprinkle each serving with some of the reserved toasted almonds.

TIP:

If your almonds have skins, they will need to be blanched and peeled. Place the almonds in a small saucepan with enough water to completely cover them. Bring to a boil and simmer for 1 to 2 minutes. Drain in a colander and cool. For rapid cooling, rinse the almonds under cold running tap water. Pinch the almonds between your thumb and index finger. The skins will slip off easily. To grind the almonds after blanching them, pat them dry or let them air dry in a single layer on a clean tea towel. When they are dry, grind them in a food processor fitted with a metal blade.

285

NAVY BEAN SOUP

Makes about 1½ quarts

1. Combine the water, onions, carrots, potato, celery, garlic, basil, and bay leaf in a large saucepan or Dutch oven and bring to a boil.
2. Cover, reduce heat to medium-low, and simmer until the vegetables are tender, about 20 minutes. Remove the bay leaf and stir in the tomato sauce and olive oil.
3. Combine 1 cup of the soup and 1½ cups of the beans (reserve the remaining 1½ cups of beans) in a blender and process until smooth. Pour this mixture into the soup pot along with the reserved beans. Stir in the parsley, if using, and season with salt and pepper to taste. Simmer over medium heat until hot, about 5 minutes.

3½ cups water

2 cups chopped onion

2 medium carrots, thinly sliced (or diced)

1 medium potato, peeled and diced

1 stalk celery, sliced

½ teaspoon minced garlic

½ teaspoon dried basil

1 whole bay leaf

1 cup tomato sauce (or ⅓ cup tomato paste blended with ⅔ cup water)

2 tablespoons extra-virgin olive oil

3 cups cooked navy beans, rinsed and drained

1 to 2 tablespoons minced fresh parsley (optional)

Salt and ground black pepper to taste

FRENCH ONION SOUP

Makes about 1½ quarts

A delectable classic that's amazingly simple to prepare.

1. Heat the oil in a 4½-quart saucepan or Dutch oven over a medium-high burner. Add the onions and garlic, reduce the heat to medium, and sauté for 5 minutes.
2. Stir in the flour, mixing well. Then stir in the water and tamari, and bring to a boil. Reduce the heat to low, cover, and simmer until the onions are tender, about 20 minutes.
3. Just before serving, place a slice of French bread or some croutons in the bottom of the soup bowls. Ladle the soup on top and serve.

1 tablespoon extra-virgin olive oil

2 large (or 3 medium) onions, sliced or chopped

1 tablespoon minced garlic

¼ cup whole-wheat pastry flour

4 cups water

¼ cup tamari

French bread, 1 slice per serving (or ¼ cup croutons per serving)

PICKLE, TAHINI, AND TOMATO SANDWICHES

Makes 2 sandwiches

A funny-sounding name for a very tasty sandwich.

Spread one side of each slice of bread with some of the tahini. Over two of the slices, layer the pickle, tomato, and onion slices. Sprinkle each layer with salt and pepper. Top with the lettuce leaves and remaining bread slices, tahini-side in.

4   slices whole-grain bread, toasted if desired

2   tablespoons tahini

2   large leaves romaine or leaf lettuce

1   medium tomato, thickly sliced

2   thin slices mild onion

2   medium dill pickles, thinly sliced lengthwise

Salt and ground black pepper to taste

BEAN BURRITOS

1. Place all the filling ingredients in a medium saucepan and bring to a boil. Reduce heat to medium and simmer uncovered for 5 minutes, stirring occasionally. Remove the saucepan from the heat and mash the beans slightly with a fork or potato masher. Cover to keep warm and set aside.

2. Warm the tortillas by placing one at a time in a dry skillet over medium heat. Warm for about 1 minute, or just until the tortilla is heated. Immediately remove the tortilla from the skillet, and lay it on a flat surface. Layer the tortillas one on top of the other after they are warmed. Cover the tortillas with a clean tea towel to lock in the heat while the remainder are warmed.

3. Spoon ¼ of the bean mixture onto each of the tortillas, placing it in a strip along one side, slightly off center. Add your favorite toppings, and roll the tortillas around the filling.

4 whole-wheat flour tortillas (lard-free)

BEAN FILLING

1½ cups soft-cooked pinto beans, drained

½ cup tomato sauce

¼ cup finely chopped bell pepper (red or green)

1 teaspoon chili powder

¼ teaspoon garlic powder

¼ teaspoon dried oregano

¼ teaspoon ground cumin

Several drops Tabasco sauce, to taste

TOPPING OPTIONS

Lettuce

Tomato

Cilantro (fresh only)

Black olives

Scallions

Tofu sour cream (see p. 310)

Onion

Avocado

CURRIED TOFU SALAD SANDWICHES

Makes 2 sandwiches

A quick lunch or light dinner that curry lovers will adore.

1. Combine the mayonnaise and curry powder in a medium mixing bowl. Stir in the pineapple and raisins. Carefully fold in the tofu cubes, mixing them in gently but thoroughly.
2. Spread the tofu mixture equally over two slices of the bread or stuff ¼ of the mixture into each of the pita pockets. Top with lettuce and serve.

¼ cup egg- and dairy-free mayonnaise

¾ to 1 teaspoon curry powder (or to taste)

1 8-ounce can unsweetened crushed pineapple, drained

2 tablespoons raisins

½ pound firm regular tofu, steamed or simmered in water for 10 minutes, then cooled, and cut into ¼-inch cubes

4 slices whole-grain bread (or 2 whole-wheat pita breads, cut in half and spread apart to form 4 pockets)

½ cup leaf lettuce or romaine lettuce, sliced into thin strips

SLICED SEITAN SANDWICHES WITH PEPPERCORN RANCH SLAW

Makes 2 sandwiches, or 4 half-sandwiches

This sandwich is a vegetarian spin-off of the Mediterranean gyro.

1. Combine the slaw vegetables in a large mixing bowl.
2. Combine the next 6 ingredients in a small bowl or measuring cup to make the Peppercorn Ranch Dressing. Pour over the slaw vegetables, and toss gently until well combined. Add the sliced seitan, and toss again gently.
3. Stuff each pita half with ¼ of the seitan-slaw mixture. Serve at once.

SLAW

1½ cups green cabbage, finely shredded

½ cup cucumber, finely diced (peel if waxed or thick-skinned, and remove seeds if they are very large)

1 small carrot, pared and shredded

PEPPERCORN RANCH DRESSING

¼ cup egg- and dairy-free mayonnaise

½ teaspoon dried tarragon leaves

¼ teaspoon dried dill weed

⅛ to ¼ teaspoon coarsely ground black pepper (or to taste)

⅛ teaspoon onion powder

⅛ teaspoon garlic powder

½ cup seitan, drained, patted dry, and sliced into thin strips

2 whole-wheat pita breads, cut in half and spread apart to form 4 pockets

RED RIBBON RICE

Serves 4 to 6 as a side dish

This rice dish is fragrant, festive, and easy to prepare, making it ideal for every day or for entertaining.

1. Place the water, raisins, nutritional yeast, rosemary, garlic, and salt in a 2-quart or larger saucepan and bring to a boil.
2. Stir in rice, cover, and simmer until almost all of the liquid has been absorbed, about 15 to 20 minutes.
3. Remove from heat, stir up the rice so that the drier kernels on top are mixed with the wetter ones on the bottom. Cover and let stand for 5 minutes.
4. Stir in bell pepper, walnuts, and oil, and toss gently until evenly distributed.

1½ cups water

½ cup raisins

1 tablespoon nutritional yeast flakes

1 teaspoon fresh rosemary (or ¼ teaspoon dried rosemary)

1 teaspoon minced garlic

½ teaspoon salt

1 cup white basmati rice

1 small red bell pepper, sliced into matchsticks

½ cup coarsely chopped walnuts

1 tablespoon organic flaxseed oil (or extra-virgin olive oil)

SUMMER SQUASH AND RED PEPPER MEDLEY

Serves 4 as a side dish

Colorful seasonal vegetables require little cooking and minimal seasoning yet make delicious, eye-appealing fare.

1. Heat the oil in a large skillet or wok over medium heat. Add the garlic and sauté for 1 minute. Add the zucchini and squash and sauté for 5 minutes. Stir in the red bell pepper and continue to sauté until all the vegetables are tender, about 5 minutes longer.
2. Sprinkle in the tamari and lemon juice and toss until the vegetables are evenly coated.

1 tablespoon extra-virgin olive oil

½ teaspoon minced garlic

2 large zucchini, cut into thick matchsticks

2 large yellow summer squash, cut into thick matchsticks

½ cup finely diced red bell pepper

1 tablespoon tamari

1 tablespoon fresh lemon juice

BROCCOLI CHEESE GRITS

Serves 2 as a main dish or breakfast; serves 4 as a side dish

Although some might think it strange, I love hot polenta for breakfast. It also makes an interesting main meal or side dish. Nutritional yeast flakes add cheeselike undertones, while broccoli adds flavor, nutrition, and beautiful flecks of green. Do not be tempted to substitute cornmeal, as you will not have good results. Use only the more coarsely ground corn grits, which can be found in natural-food stores.

- 2 cups water
- ½ cup yellow (or white) corn grits
- ½ to 1 cup finely chopped broccoli
- 2 tablespoons nutritional yeast flakes
- 2 teaspoons extra-virgin olive oil
- 2 teaspoons organic flaxseed oil (or additional olive oil)
- ½ teaspoon salt

1. Combine the water, and broccoli in a heavy-bottomed saucepan and bring to a boil. Simmer for 5 minutes.
2. Remove from heat and stir in the grits with a long-handled wooden spoon. Return to a boil. Reduce heat to low, cover and cook, stirring occasionally, for 20 minutes.
3. Stir well, add remaining ingredients, and mix thoroughly.

TIP:
If the polenta sticks to the bottom of your saucepan, use a flame tamer (also called a heat diffuser) underneath.

LEMON AND GARLIC BROCCOLI

Serves 2 to 4 as a side dish

It doesn't take much effort to turn versatile broccoli into something really special, and this quick and easy recipe does exactly that.

4 cups broccoli flowerets

3 tablespoons fresh lemon juice

1 tablespoon extra-virgin olive oil

½ to 1 teaspoon minced garlic, to taste

Pinch of crushed red chili peppers, to taste

Steam the broccoli until tender. Transfer to a medium bowl. Combine the lemon juice, oil, garlic, and crushed red chili peppers in a small bowl or measuring cup and whisk together until blended. Pour over the broccoli and toss until evenly coated. Serve hot, warm, or chilled.

BRUSSELS SPROUTS IN SWEET MUSTARD SAUCE

Serves 4 as a side dish

If brussels sprouts aren't on your list of favorite vegetables, try this tempting recipe— it could very well change your mind. If you do love brussels sprouts, you'll definitely want to add this to your repertoire.

1 pound fresh brussels sprouts, trimmed and quartered

2 tablespoons extra-virgin olive oil

1 tablespoon fresh lemon juice

2 teaspoons Dijon mustard

2 teaspoons sugar

1. Bring a large pot of water to a rolling boil. Add the brussels sprouts and cook until tender. Drain well.
2. Combine the oil, lemon juice, mustard, and sugar in a small bowl or measuring cup. Whisk them together until blended. Pour over the brussels sprouts and toss until evenly coated.

MARINATED CARROT STICKS

Serves 6 to 8 as a side dish

Serve marinated carrot sticks as a special appetizer, side dish, or tasty addition to a vegetarian antipasto. They are also great to keep in the fridge for a no-fuss, no-muss snack.

8 to 10 carrots, cut into sticks about 2½ inches long by ½ inch thick

⅓ cup red wine vinegar

¼ cup extra-virgin olive oil

½ teaspoon minced garlic

Generous pinch of salt

1. Place an inch of water in a large saucepan and bring to a boil. Add the carrots, cover, and cook over medium heat until tender-crisp, about 6 to 8 minutes. Drain and transfer to a bowl.

2. Combine the remaining ingredients in a small bowl or measuring cup and whisk them together until blended. Pour over the carrots and toss until evenly coated. Cover tightly and refrigerate several hours or overnight, tossing again once or twice. Bring to room temperature before serving. Drain or serve with a slotted spoon.

MAHVELOUS MILLET LOAF

Serves 8

Millet is a highly digestible and very versatile grain. Although it can be made fluffy and pilaflike, when it is cooked with abundant water millet becomes soft and tender with a texture similar to polenta. It makes an ideal foundation for a meatless loaf.

1. Oil a large loaf pan or mist it with nonstick cooking spray. Set aside.
2. Rinse the millet well and place it in a large saucepan along with the water, onions, carrots, celery, salt, garlic, and thyme. Bring to a boil.
3. Cover and reduce the heat to medium-low. Simmer for 30 minutes.
4. Remove from the heat and let stand 10 minutes. Stir in the oil and nuts or seeds and mix well. Spoon the mixture into the prepared loaf pan, packing it down firmly. Place on a cooling rack and allow the loaf to rest in the pan at room temperature for 15 minutes. Carefully turn the loaf out of the pan onto a cutting board or serving platter. Cut into slices and serve.

TIP:
To toast the walnuts, cashews, or sunflower seeds, place them in a small dry skillet over medium heat. Stir constantly until golden brown and fragrant.

- 1 cup millet
- 2½ cups water
- 1 cup finely chopped onions
- 1 cup finely chopped (or shredded) carrots
- 1 cup finely diced celery
- 1¼ teaspoons salt
- ½ teaspoon minced garlic
- ½ teaspoon dried thyme
- 2 tablespoons extra-virgin olive oil
- ½ to 1 cup chopped pistachios, toasted walnuts, cashews, or sunflower seeds

LEAFY GREEN PIZZA WITH BASIL AND OLIVES

Serves 4 to 6

Even people who might typically shy away from greens will gobble up this pizza without coaxing. Sliced fresh tomatoes make a tasty side dish.

1. Preheat the oven to 400 degrees F. Place the crust on a dry baking sheet (or pizza pan or baking stone) and set aside.

2. Heat the oil in a very large skillet and sauté the garlic in it for about a minute. Add the kale, cover, and cook over medium heat, stirring often, until fairly tender, about 8 to 10 minutes. Add the olives, tomatoes (if using), basil, and salt and remove the skillet from the heat.

3. Distribute the kale mixture evenly over the crust. Sprinkle the nutritional yeast evenly over the top. Bake until the crust is crisp, about 10 to 15 minutes. Watch closely so the topping doesn't burn.

PIZZA CRUST *(Your Choice)*

1. loaf French or Italian bread (16 to 20 inches long), cut in half width- and lengthwise

1. French baguette (18 to 22 inches long), cut in half width- and lengthwise

1. prebaked pizza shell (15-inch diameter), thawed to room temperature

3. pita breads (6-inch diameter), sliced around the outer edge to form 6 equal rounds

TOPPING

4. tablespoons extra-virgin olive oil

1. tablespoon minced garlic

6. cups chopped fresh kale (stems removed; firmly packed)

⅓ cup oil-cured ripe olives, pitted and coarsely chopped

⅓ cup sun-dried tomatoes packed in oil, drained and chopped (optional)

⅓ cup chopped fresh basil (or 1 tablespoon dried basil)

¼ to ½ teaspoon salt, to taste

¼ cup nutritional yeast flakes

ROASTED VEGETABLE PIZZA WITH TOMATO-TINGED TOFU

Serves 4 to 6

This is a long name for a very simple dish. French bread is sliced in half, spread with a well-seasoned tofu pâté, topped with your choice of seasonal vegetables, and baked to golden perfection. Now who said healthful food is boring?

1. Preheat the oven to 450 degrees F. Place the crust on a dry baking sheet (or pizza pan or baking stone) and set aside.

2. Place all the pâté ingredients in a food processor and blend into a smooth paste. Spread the mixture evenly over the crust.

3. Toss the vegetables with the olive oil until they are evenly coated. Distribute the vegetables evenly over the top of the pâté and press them in lightly (so they don't fall off).

4. Bake until the vegetables are lightly browned, the tofu is hot, and the crust is crisp, about 10 to 15 minutes.

PIZZA CRUST *(Your Choice)*

1 loaf French or Italian bread (16 to 20 inches long), cut in half width- and lengthwise

1 French baguette (18 to 22 inches long), cut in half width- and lengthwise

1 prebaked pizza shell (15-inch diameter), thawed to room temperature

3 pita breads (6-inch diameter), sliced around the outer edge to form 6 equal rounds

TOFU PÂTÉ

½ pound firm regular tofu, rinsed, patted dry, and crumbled

2 tablespoons tomato paste

2 tablespoons extra-virgin olive oil

1 tablespoon tamari

1 teaspoon ground fennel (or dried basil)

1 teaspoon dried oregano

1 teaspoon minced garlic

⅛ to ¼ teaspoon cayenne pepper

Salt to taste

Ground black pepper to taste

TIP:

Good vegetable choices include (but are not limited to) onion, zucchini, red or green bell pepper, roasted red peppers, mushrooms, water-packed artichoke hearts, scallion, shallots, firm fresh tomatoes, ripe olives, shredded carrot, and capers.

VEGGIES

2 cups very thinly sliced (or finely chopped) mixed vegetables (see tip)

1 tablespoon extra-virgin olive oil

SAVORY BAKED TOFU

Serves 2 to 4

This dish requires advance planning, but it's so easy to prepare it's almost ridiculous. The baked tofu makes a great dinner entrée as well as a scrumptious sandwich filling. You can also slice leftovers into strips or cubes and use it to top salads, toss with pasta, or stir into cooked rice. If you use tofu that was processed with calcium sulfate, this dish will be an excellent source of calcium. It's a delicious and easy way to eat healthfully!

½ pound firm regular tofu, rinsed and patted dry

½ to 1 cup Italian dressing

Seasoned salt or salt-free herb seasoning (optional)

1. Cut the tofu into ½-inch-thick slices. Place them in a ceramic bowl and pour the dressing over them, using as much as necessary to cover the tofu completely. Turn the tofu slices over so that each side is coated with the dressing. Cover the bowl and let the tofu marinate in the refrigerator for a minimum of 6 to 8 hours.

2. Preheat the oven to 350 degrees F. Lightly oil a baking sheet. Remove the tofu from the marinade, letting the excess dressing drain off. Arrange the tofu in a single layer on the baking sheet and sprinkle lightly with seasoned salt or salt-free herb seasoning, if desired. Bake for 20 minutes. Serve hot or cold.

TIP:

This recipe is very easy to double, triple, or quadruple. It's a good, quick entrée for company because once it's marinated and in the oven it requires no attention. It also makes a terrific addition to salads of all kinds—pasta, potato, or grain salads—so it's perfect for potlucks and picnics.

IGOR'S SPECIAL

Serves 2

This quick pasta dish was contributed by Paula Barry, who learned the recipe from her friend Igor. Having relied on it on numerous hectic occasions, I can attest that this recipe is not only delicious, it can be on the table in 20 minutes!

1. Cook the pasta until it is al dente. Do not drain. Remove the pot from the heat, and add the broccoli flowerets. Cover with a lid and let the pasta and broccoli sit for 5 to 8 minutes. Drain well in a colander.

2 While the pasta and broccoli are sitting, combine the remaining ingredients *except the salt or tamari* in a large bowl. Add the drained pasta and broccoli and toss gently but thoroughly. Taste; add more vinegar if you like a sharper flavor. Season with salt or tamari. Toss again and serve.

TIP:

This is a great last-minute company dish as it is easily doubled and takes practically no time to prepare.

6   ounces pasta (any kind, your choice)

2   cups bite-size broccoli flowerets

1   large ripe tomato (or 2 to 3 ripe roma tomatoes), chopped

¼   cup chopped red onion or sliced scallions

¼   cup coarsely chopped walnuts

1   tablespoon fresh lemon juice

1   tablespoon vinegar (red wine or balsamic), or more to taste

1   tablespoon extra-virgin olive oil

¼   teaspoon minced garlic

¼   teaspoon curry powder, or more to taste

Dash of cayenne pepper

Dash of ground black pepper

Salt (or tamari) to taste

QUINOA PRIMAVERA

Serves 2 to 3

Because quinoa cooks so quickly, this grain-based entrée can be on the table in less than 30 minutes.

1. Place the water in a medium saucepan and bring to a boil. Stir in the quinoa. Cover with a lid and reduce the heat to low. Simmer for 15 to 18 minutes. Remove from the heat and scatter the peas on top of the grain; do not stir. Replace the lid and let rest for 8 minutes.

2. While the quinoa rests, place the olive oil in a large skillet or wok over medium-high heat. When the oil is hot, add the carrot, zucchini, red bell pepper, leek, and garlic. Stir-fry for about 8 minutes or until the carrot is tender-crisp. Stir in the quinoa and peas along with the dill. Toss together until thoroughly combined. Heat over medium heat, tossing constantly, until the peas are heated through, about 2 minutes. Season with salt and pepper.

1¼ cups water

½ cup quinoa, rinsed well

1 cup frozen green peas, thawed under hot tap water and drained

1 tablespoon extra-virgin olive oil

1 medium carrot, thinly sliced on the diagonal

1 medium zucchini, thinly sliced on the diagonal

1 small red bell pepper, chopped

1 large leek, thinly sliced (use only the white bulb and tender green portion)

½ teaspoon minced garlic

1 tablespoon chopped fresh dill (or 1 teaspoon dried dill)

Salt and ground black pepper to taste

BAKED POTATOES FLORENTINE

Serves 4 to 8

This satisfying potato entrée with its luscious herb and spinach topping will undoubtedly make you forget about dairy sour cream forever.

1. Combine the tofu, parsley, olive oil, onion, dill, tarragon, garlic, salt, and pepper in a food processor fitted with a metal blade and blend until smooth and creamy. Transfer to a medium bowl.
2. Cook the spinach according to the package directions. Drain in a wire mesh strainer or colander, pressing firmly with a fork or the back of a spoon to extract as much liquid as possible. Stir into the tofu mixture along with the water chestnuts, if using, and scallions. Adjust salt and pepper, if necessary.
3. Split the hot baked potatoes in half, fluff the flesh gently with a fork, and spoon the spinach mixture on top. Garnish with a light dusting of paprika.

TIP:

To bake potatoes, first scrub them well. Preheat the oven to 375 degrees F. Place the potatoes directly on the center rack of the oven and bake for 1 to 1½ hours or until soft when gently squeezed (use an oven mitt!).

4	hot baked potatoes
1½	cups silken tofu, firmly packed
⅓	cup minced fresh parsley
2 to 3	tablespoons extra-virgin olive oil
2	tablespoons minced onion
1	teaspoon dried dill
1	teaspoon dried tarragon
½	teaspoon minced garlic
½	teaspoon salt (or to taste)
	Ground black pepper to taste
1	10-ounce package frozen, chopped spinach, prepared according to package directions
½	cup sliced water chestnuts, quartered (optional)
¼	cup thinly sliced scallions
	Paprika for garnish

FARMHOUSE STEW | *Serves 4*

Old-fashioned beef-stew flavor with a new-fangled twist—no beef!

1. Place the potatoes, carrots, broth or water, celery, and bay leaves in a 4½-quart saucepan or Dutch oven. Bring to a boil, then reduce the heat to medium. Cover and simmer, stirring occasionally, until the vegetables are tender, about 20 minutes.
2. Meanwhile, place the oil in a large skillet over medium-high heat. Add the onion and sauté for 8 minutes or until almost tender. Add the mushrooms and continue to sauté, stirring often, until tender, about 4 to 6 minutes longer.
3. Remove the skillet from the heat. Stir in the flour and mix well. Then stir in the tahini and mix well. Gradually stir in the ½ cup water and tamari, and mix vigorously until the sauce is smooth. Stir this mixture into the hot cooked vegetables and their liquid and mix well.
4. Stir in the seitan and bring the stew to a boil, stirring almost constantly. Reduce the heat to medium and continue to stir and simmer the stew just until the sauce thickens, about 3 to 5 minutes. Remove the bay leaves and season with salt and pepper. Ladle into bowls and serve hot.

4 cups diced potatoes (thin-skinned or peeled)

4 large carrots, sliced in half lengthwise and cut into 1-inch chunks

2 cups vegetable broth (or water)

2 stalks celery, finely chopped

2 bay leaves

1 tablespoon extra-virgin olive oil

1 cup chopped onions

2 cups sliced mushrooms

2 tablespoons whole-wheat pastry flour

2 tablespoons tahini

½ cup water

3 tablespoons tamari

2 cups seitan chunks

Salt and ground black pepper to taste

SAUCY BEANS AND FRANKS

Serves 4

Children love this dish because it's fun to eat and tastes terrific. Adults love it because it's a quick, nutritious, last-minute entrée. Serve it with whole-grain rolls or biscuits and coleslaw.

Combine all the ingredients in a 4½-quart saucepan or Dutch oven. Place over medium heat, stirring occasionally, until hot and bubbly.

3 cups cooked beans, drained (pinto, white beans, or any other bean you prefer)

⅔ cup ketchup

4 vegan hot dogs, cooked according to package directions and sliced into ¼-inch rounds

2 tablespoons tamari

2 tablespoons light molasses (or pure maple syrup)

2 teaspoons vinegar (brown-rice, balsamic, or red-wine vinegar)

1 teaspoon onion powder

½ teaspoon dry mustard

Several drops liquid hickory smoke (optional)

TOFU RICOTTA

Makes about 1½ cups

Use this versatile filling to stuff pasta shells, lasagna, or manicotti, or toss it with pasta or spaghetti squash and bake in a casserole. For a different flavor, add chopped spinach or fresh basil and some vegan soy Parmesan.

½	pound regular tofu (firm)
2	tablespoons extra-virgin olive oil
1½	teaspoons nutritional yeast flakes (optional)
½	teaspoon dried basil
½	teaspoon dried oregano
½	teaspoon garlic powder
½	teaspoon onion powder
½	teaspoon salt

1. Steam the tofu for 2 to 5 minutes. Let cool, then pat dry and crumble into a medium mixing bowl.
2. Add the remaining ingredients and toss until well combined. Taste and adjust seasonings, if necessary. Use immediately or store in a covered container in the refrigerator for future use.

ALMOND MAYONNAISE

Makes about 1 cup

This spread offers a very rich and creamy alternative to commercial mayonnaise. It's also great for soy-sensitive children and adults, since most prepared mayonnaise substitutes are tofu-based.

Grind the almonds in a blender. Add the water or milk, nutritional yeast flakes, salt, and garlic powder and process until fairly smooth. With the blender on low, add the olive oil and flaxseed oil in a slow, steady stream. Stop and start as needed in order to stir the mixture and scrape down the sides of the blender jar. Add the lemon juice and vinegar and process until thick and creamy. Store in a tightly covered container in the refrigerator. It will keep 10 to 14 days.

¼ cup blanched almonds

¼ cup water (or plain nondairy milk)

½ teaspoon nutritional yeast flakes

¼ teaspoon salt

¼ teaspoon garlic powder

⅓ cup extra-virgin olive oil

2 tablespoons organic flaxseed oil (or additional olive oil)

2 tablespoons fresh lemon juice

½ teaspoon apple-cider vinegar

VEGAN MAYONNAISE

Makes about 1⅓ cups

Use this egg- and dairy-free mayonnaise in place of traditional mayonnaise for all your favorite recipes.

Combine all the ingredients in a food processor fitted with a metal blade, or in a blender, and process several minutes until very smooth and creamy. Use at once or store in the refrigerator for up to 10 days.

1½ cups silken tofu (firm), crumbled

1 tablespoon extra-virgin olive oil

1 tablespoon organic flaxseed oil (or additional olive oil)

2 teaspoons fresh lemon juice

2 teaspoons apple-cider vinegar

1½ teaspoons sugar (or 2 teaspoons brown-rice syrup)

Heaping ½ teaspoon salt

½ teaspoon prepared yellow mustard

TOFU SOUR CREAM

Makes about 1½ cups

Use this luscious dairy-free topping wherever you would typically use dairy sour cream. It's magnificent tasting and so simple to prepare.

Combine all the ingredients in a blender or food processor fitted with a metal blade and process until creamy. Chill before serving.

1½ cups silken tofu, crumbled and firmly packed

2 tablespoons extra-virgin olive oil

2 teaspoons fresh lemon juice

2 teaspoons apple-cider vinegar

½ teaspoon sugar

½ teaspoon salt

FRUIT-BUTTER BARS

Makes 12 to 16 bars

This old-fashioned favorite is easy to make. It's a lunch-box staple, a wholesome snack, and a welcome dessert.

1½ cups whole-wheat pastry flour

1½ cups quick-cooking rolled oats (not instant)

¼ cup sugar

½ teaspoon baking soda

¼ teaspoon salt

½ cup pure maple syrup

¼ cup canola oil

1½ cups thick fruit butter (apple, prune, or peach)

1. Preheat the oven to 350 degrees F. Lightly oil the sides and bottom of a glass baking pan 8 inches square and 2 inches deep, or mist it with nonstick cooking spray.
2. To make the crust, place the flour, oats, sugar, baking soda, and salt in a large mixing bowl, and stir them together until well combined. In a small mixing bowl, stir together the maple syrup and canola oil. Pour into the flour-oat mixture and mix thoroughly until everything is evenly moistened. The mixture will be crumbly.
3. Press half this mixture evenly into the prepared baking pan, packing it down very firmly. Carefully spread the fruit butter evenly over this base. Sprinkle the rest of the flour-oat mixture evenly over the fruit butter, and pat it down lightly.
4. Bake for 20 to 25 minutes, or until lightly browned. Cool on a wire rack, and slice into bars or squares.

THE ULTIMATE CHOCOLATE-CHIP COOKIE

Makes about 32 two-inch cookies

One bite and chocolate-chip-cookie lovers will know they have met their match!

1. Preheat the oven to 350 degrees F. Line two baking sheets with parchment paper. Set aside.
2. Place the oats, flour, nuts, chocolate chips, salt, and baking soda in a large mixing bowl. Stir with a wire whisk.
3. Place the oil, maple syrup, water, and vanilla in a small mixing bowl and beat vigorously with a wire whisk until emulsified. Stir into the oat-flour mixture, mixing just until everything is evenly moistened. Let sit 5 minutes.
4. Drop slightly rounded tablespoons of dough onto the prepared baking sheets, about 1 inch apart. The dough will be crumbly. Flatten with your hand to ⅓-inch thick. Smooth the edges to make each cookie uniformly round, gently pressing the dough so that the cookies hold together.
5. Bake *one sheet at a time* on the center shelf of the oven until cookies are lightly brown, about 18 minutes. Transfer to a cooling rack and cool completely. Store in an airtight container in the refrigerator.

1½ cups quick-cooking rolled oats (not instant)

1 cup whole-wheat pastry flour

1 cup walnuts, lightly toasted and chopped (see tip)

1 cup semisweet vegan chocolate chips

½ teaspoon salt

¼ teaspoon baking soda

½ cup canola oil

½ cup pure maple syrup

2 tablespoons water

2 teaspoons vanilla extract

TIP:

To toast the walnuts, preheat the oven to 350 degrees F. Spread the nuts in a single layer on a dry baking sheet. Bake on the center shelf of the oven until fragrant and lightly browned, about 8 to 10 minutes.

The cookies taste best after they have been chilled in the refrigerator.

APPLE COBBLER

Serves 4 to 6

This luscious fruit tart makes your "apple a day" taste especially wonderful.

1. Preheat the oven to 350 degrees F. Lightly oil a glass baking pan 8 inches square by 2 inches deep and set aside.
2. For the topping, combine the flour, oats, and baking powder in a medium mixing bowl. Place the apple-juice concentrate and oil in a small measuring cup, and whisk them together. Pour into the oat-flour mixture, and cut in using a pastry blender or fork until crumbly. Set aside.
3. For the filling, place the apple slices and raisins in a large mixing bowl. Sprinkle with the lemon juice and toss gently.
4. Place the juice concentrate, flour, and cinnamon in a small measuring cup, and beat them together using a wire whisk or a fork until the mixture is very smooth. Pour over the apples and raisins, and toss until the fruit is evenly coated.
5. Spoon the fruit and any liquid remaining in the bowl into the prepared baking pan. Crumble the reserved topping evenly over the top. Bake for 30 minutes or until the top is golden brown and the apples are fork tender. Serve hot, warm, room temperature, or chilled.

TOPPING

- ⅔ cup whole-wheat pastry flour
- ⅔ cup quick-cooking rolled oats (not instant)
- ½ teaspoon double-acting nonaluminum baking powder
- ¼ cup frozen apple-juice concentrate
- 2 tablespoons canola oil

FILLING

- 4 medium Granny Smith apples, peeled and sliced
- ⅓ cup raisins
- 1½ tablespoons fresh lemon juice
- ¼ cup frozen apple-juice concentrate
- 2 tablespoons whole-wheat pastry flour
- ½ teaspoon ground cinnamon

TIP:

For an extra special dessert, top each serving with a scoop of dairy-free vanilla frozen dessert.

RED DEVIL CAKE

Serves 9 to 12

This cake has a secret ingredient—blended beets! Despite its wholesomeness, you'll be amazed how sinfully delicious it is!

2 cups whole-wheat pastry flour

1 cup sugar

½ cup cocoa powder

2 teaspoons double-acting nonaluminum baking powder

2 teaspoons baking soda

½ teaspoon salt

2 tablespoons flaxseeds

⅓ cup water

1 cup diced cooked beets

1 cup water

⅓ cup canola oil

2 teaspoons apple-cider vinegar

2 teaspoons vanilla extract

1. Preheat the oven to 350 degrees F. Lightly oil the bottom and sides of an 8-inch square baking pan or mist it with nonstick cooking spray.

2. Place the flour, sugar, cocoa powder, baking powder, baking soda, and salt in a medium mixing bowl and stir them with a wire whisk until well combined.

3. Place the flaxseeds in a dry blender and grind them into a powder. Add the ⅓ cup water and blend until a gummy mixture is achieved, about 30 seconds. Add the beets, 1 cup water, canola oil, vinegar, and vanilla, and process until frothy and well blended, about 1 to 2 minutes. Pour into the flour mixture and mix just until everything is evenly moistened.

4. Quickly spoon the batter into the prepared pan. Bake until a toothpick inserted in the center comes out clean, about 35 to 40 minutes. Cool on a rack for at least 30 minutes before serving. When completely cool, frost with Creamy Fudge Frosting (see p. 315). Store the frosted cake tightly covered in the refrigerator.

CREAMY FUDGE FROSTING

Makes about 1½ cups

1. Process the tofu and maple syrup in a food processor until smooth and creamy, about 2 minutes. Transfer to a small, heavy saucepan. Add the chocolate chips and stir to combine.
2. Warm over very low heat, stirring constantly while scraping the sides and bottom of the pan, until the chips have melted completely. Stir well to thoroughly blend in the chocolate. Remove from the heat and stir in the vanilla.
3. Transfer to a covered container and refrigerate several hours until well chilled. Stir again before using.

1 cup silken tofu, crumbled

3 tablespoons pure maple syrup

1 cup semisweet vegan chocolate chips

½ teaspoon vanilla extract

KEEPSAKE BROWNIES

Serves 12 to 16

Oil or nonstick cooking spray

Cocoa powder

2 tablespoons flaxseeds

1 cup water

4 squares (1 ounce each) unsweetened baking chocolate

½ cup canola oil

1½ cups sugar

1 teaspoon vanilla extract

¾ cup whole-wheat pastry flour

½ cup chopped walnuts (optional)

1. Preheat the oven to 350 degrees F. Oil the bottom and sides of an 8-inch-square baking pan and dust it lightly with cocoa powder. Tap the pan on the countertop firmly on all sides to distribute the cocoa evenly. Alternatively, mist the pan with nonstick cooking spray.

2. Place the flaxseeds in a dry blender and grind them into a powder. Add the water and blend until a gummy mixture is achieved, about 30 seconds. Set aside.

3. Melt the chocolate in a heavy 2-quart saucepan over low heat. Remove from the heat and stir in the oil and then the sugar with a wooden spoon. Mix vigorously until well blended. Stir in the vanilla extract and mix again. Pour in the reserved flaxseed mixture and beat well. Add the flour and stir until the batter is thoroughly blended and smooth. Stir in the walnuts, if using.

4. Pour the batter into the prepared pan (scrape it out with a rubber spatula to get every last bit). If necessary, ease the batter into the corners and edges of the pan so that it is evenly distributed. Bake for 20 to 25 minutes for fudgey brownies, or 30 minutes for cakelike brownies. *Do not overbake!* Cool before serving (if you can wait that long!). Store leftovers tightly covered at room temperature or in the refrigerator.

THE VEGAN LIFELINE:

RESOURCES AND ORGANIZATIONS

This resource guide is an introduction to a number of organizations, publications, and mail-order sources that can provide assistance on the vegan journey. Some of the organizations have their own publications; most offer pamphlets and educational materials; and some have videos for rent or sale. Many of the organizations also have Websites, and there is an exhaustive network of additional vegan resources on-line. Just do a comprehensive search on key words such as *vegan* or *animal rights* to find current Web addresses. Most will have links to many more great sites.

Organizations

The American Anti-Vivisection Society (AAVS)
801 Old York Road, No. 204
Jenkintown, PA 19046
Phone: (215) 887-0816
Fax: (215) 887-2088

Dedicated to the elimination of animal use in research, product testing, and education. Offers pamphlets, videos, and educational materials.

American Vegan Society (AVS)
P.O. Box 369
Malaga, NJ 08328-0908
Phone: (856) 694-2887
Fax: (856) 694-2288

A nonprofit, educational, membership organization teaching the vegan way of life. Publishes the quarterly magazine *Ahimsa*. Offers books, pamphlets, videotapes, and audiotapes by mail. Coordinates an annual vegan conference featuring prominent leaders in animal rights, nutrition, economics, environmentalism, and other concerns related to the vegan cause.

Animal Legal Defense Fund (ALDF)
127 Fourth Street
Petaluma, CA 94952-3005
Phone: (707) 769-7771
Fax: (707) 769-0785

A nationwide network of attorneys dedicated to protecting and promoting animal rights.

Association of Veterinarians for Animal Rights (AVAR)
P.O. Box 208
Davis, CA 95617-0208
Phone: (530) 759-8106
Fax: (530) 759-8116

Educates the public and veterinarians about animal abuse, specifically the use of animals in veterinary education and a variety of companion animal issues. Goal is to constantly challenge the way veterinarians are trained and to raise the consciousness of the profession. Has pamphlets and leaflets available for the general public with regard to companion-animal issues.

Center for Compassionate Living (CCL)
P.O. Box 1209
Blue Hill, ME 04614
Phone: (207) 374-8808
Fax: (207) 374-8851

Offers training, consulting, workshops, and outdoor experiences for people who want to help the planet and all its inhabitants. Launched the first humane-education certification program in the United States.

Culture & Animals Foundation (CAF)
3509 Eden Croft Drive
Raleigh, NC 27612
Phone: (919) 782-3739
Fax: (919) 782-6464

A nonprofit cultural organization committed to fostering the growth of intellectual and artistic endeavors united by a positive concern for animals.

EarthSave International
1509 Seabright Avenue, Suite B1
Santa Cruz, CA 95062
Phone: 1-800-362-3648
Fax: (831) 423-1313

Educates people about the cumulative impact of our food choices on our health and the environment. Local action groups in many cities nationwide. Membership includes quarterly newsmagazine and local publications when applicable.

Farm Animal Reform Movement (FARM)
P.O. Box 30654
Bethesda, MD 20824
Phone: (301) 530-1737
Fax: (301) 530-5747

Works to expose and stop animal abuse and other destructive impacts of animal agriculture. Conducts several national grassroots campaigns including the Great American Meatout (March 20), World Farm Animals Day (October 2), and National Veal Ban Action (Mother's Day).

Farm Sanctuary West
P.O. Box 1065
Orland, CA 95963
Phone: (530) 865-4617

Farm Sanctuary East
P.O. Box 150
Watkins Glen, NY 14891
Phone: (607) 583-2225

Works to promote vegan living and stop all aspects of animal exploitation caused by the food-animal industries. Rescues abused, neglected, and abandoned farm animals, investigates and exposes abusers, and lobbies for legislative change. Provides public education and outreach. Maintains two sanctuaries where sick or injured farm animals can be rehabilitated and cared for the remainder of their natural lives. Publishes books, educational materials, and videos with graphic footage of abuses within the food animal industries. Both sanctuaries offer farm tours open to the public and sponsor a variety of educational programs, activist conferences, and events throughout the year. The New York shelter also operates a vegan bed and breakfast.

Food Not Bombs
3145 Geary Boulevard, No. 12
San Francisco, CA 94118
Phone: 1-800-884-1136

An all-volunteer peace network that provides free, hot vegan meals and political support to low-income people in North America and Europe. Local volunteers operate chapters in their communities.

The Fund for Animals
Headquarters:
200 West Fifty-seventh Street
New York, NY 10019
Phone: (212) 246-2096

For literature, videos, and further information contact:

The Fund for Animals
World Building
8121 Georgia Avenue, Suite 301
Silver Spring, MD 20910
Phone: (301) 585-2591
Fax: (301) 585-2595

Works to protect wildlife and eliminate cruelty to animals wherever, however, and whenever it occurs. Is the nation's leading antihunting organization. Offers educational materials and videos on a wide variety of animal-rights topics.

Humane Society of the United States (HSUS)
2100 L Street, NW
Washington, DC 20037
Phone: (202) 452-1100
Fax: (202) 778-6132

The nation's largest animal protection organization. Dedicated to improving the lives of animals, both domestic and wild. Provides legislative, investigative, educational, and legal support to local humane organizations, animal-control agencies, officials, educators, media, and the general public.

Institute for the Development of Earth Awareness (I.D.E.A.)
P.O. Box 124
Prince Street Station
New York, NY 10012
Phone: (212) 741-0338

An educational organization that takes a multi-issue approach to the world's problems and believes that only by recognizing the interconnectedness of all life will we realize that the fate of all life is also intertwined.

In Defense of Animals (IDA)
131 Camino Alto, Suite E
Mill Valley, CA 94941
Phone: (415) 388-9641
Fax: (415) 388-0388

Opposes the use of animals for medical or scientific research, teaching, product testing, and other areas of exploitation. Stresses nonviolent action. Acts as national coordinator for the U.S. activities of World Lab Animal Liberation Week.

National Anti-Vivisection Society (NAVS)
53 West Jackson Boulevard
Suite 1552
Chicago, IL 60604
Phone: (312) 427-6065
Toll free: 1-800-888-NAVS (6287)
Dissection Hotline: 1-800-922-FROG (3764)
Fax: (312) 427-6524

Works to abolish the use of animals for medical and scientific research, testing, and training.

New England Anti-Vivisection Society (NEAVS)
333 Washington Street, Suite 850
Boston, MA 02108
Phone: (617) 523-6020
Fax: (617) 523-7925

Presents extensive antivivisection education programs throughout New England as well as free books and materials to thousands of school libraries nationwide. Supports grassroots activism and legislative change on behalf of animals.

North American Vegetarian Society (NAVS)
P.O. Box 72
Dolgeville, NY 13329
Phone: (518) 568-7970
Fax: (518) 568-7979

A national, nonprofit educational organization dedicated to promoting the vegan-vegetarian way of life. Encourages and assists in the formation of local vegetarian groups. Originator and organizer of annual World Vegetarian Day (October 1). Publishes the quarterly magazine *Vegetarian Voice,* which includes a nationwide list of groups and contacts, merchandise offerings, and videos for sale or rental. Sponsors the annual Vegetarian Summerfest, a totally vegan event featuring premier leaders in the vegan-vegetarian, animal-rights, and environmental movements.

Peace Abbey
Strawberry Fields
Two North Main Street
Sherborn, MA 01770
Phone: (508) 650-3659

An interfaith retreat center for peacemakers from around the world. Home of Emily, the cow made famous by escaping the slaughterhouse.

Performing Animal Welfare Society (PAWS)
P.O. Box 849
Galt, CA 95632-9979
Phone: (209) 745-PAWS (7297)
Fax: (209) 745-1809

Works to protect performing animals, provide shelter for retired performing animals and unwanted "exotic" animals in need of permanent housing, and enhance the lives of captive wildlife. Conducts lobbying, litigation, and public education.

People for the Ethical Treatment of Animals (PETA)
501 Front Street
Norfolk, VA 23510
Phone: (757) 622-PETA (7382)
Fax: (757) 622-0457

Supports and defends the rights of all animals on all fronts. Has an exhaustive inventory of videos for rent and sale, books, literature, activist materials, and other merchandise.

Physicians Committee for Responsible Medicine (PCRM)
5100 Wisconsin Avenue NW, Suite 404
Washington, DC 20016
Phone: (202) 686-2210
Fax: (202) 686-2216

Promotes vegan nutrition, preventive medicine, ethical research practices, and compassionate medical policy. Membership open to both physicians and nonphysicians.

Pure Food Campaign
860 Highway 61
Little Marais, MN 55614
Activist or media inquiries: (218) 226-4164
Requests for consumer information: 1-800-253-0681
Fax: (218) 226-4157

Supports an international boycott of genetically engineered foods, and campaigns to reform school food programs.

United Poultry Concerns (UPC)
P.O. Box 150
Machipongo, VA 23405
Phone: (757) 678-7875

Promotes the compassionate and respectful treatment of domestic fowl. Offers educational literature, activist materials, books, and videos.

Vegetarian Dietitians and Nutrition Educators (VEGEDINE)
c/o George Eisman
3835 State Route 414
Burdett, NY 14818
Phone: (607) 546-7171

A support and referral group for nutrition professionals who are vegetarians or who provide services for vegetarians. Publishes the newsletter *Issues in Vegetarian Dietetics* and maintains a directory of vegetarian dietetic professionals.

Vegetarian Resource Group (VRG)
P.O. Box 1463
Baltimore, MD 21203
Phone: (410) 366-VEGE (8343)
Fax: (410) 366-8804

Promotes vegan and vegetarian nutrition. Provides education about the interrelated issues of health, nutrition, ecology, ethics, animal rights, and world hunger. Publishes a variety of books in addition to the bimonthly *Vegetarian Journal,* which is included with membership.

Vegetarian Union of North America (VUNA)
P.O. Box 9710
Washington, DC 20016

A network of vegetarian groups throughout the United States and Canada. Membership is open to vegetarian societies, other groups, and individuals. As a regional council of the International Vegetarian Union, VUNA serves as a liaison with the worldwide vegetarian movement, and VUNA members are also considered members of IVU. Mission is to promote a strong, effective, cooperative vegetarian movement throughout North America. All memberships include subscription to the quarterly VUNA newsletter and the IVU newsletter.

Mail-Order Sources

American Vegan Society (AVS)
P.O. Box 369
Malaga, NJ 08328-0908
Phone: (856) 694-2887
Fax: (856) 694-2288

Offers an extensive selection of books on vegan living, environmentalism, animal rights, pregnancy, and feeding vegan children, as well as videotapes, and audiotapes, all available by mail.

Diamond Organics
P.O. Box 2159
Freedom, CA 95019
Phone: 1-800-922-2396
Fax: 1-800-290-3683

A beautiful and impressive variety of organic fresh fruits and vegetables shipped direct.

Dixie USA, Inc.
P.O. Box 55549
Houston, TX 77255
Phone: 1-800-233-3668

Produces an extensive array of innovative soy-based food items and vegan "health food that tastes like junk food."

Gold Mine Natural Food Co.
3419 Hancock Street
San Diego, CA 92110
Phone: 1-800-475-FOOD (3663)
Fax: (619) 296-9756

A large selection of organic beans and grains, macrobiotic foods, and cooking equipment.

Heartland Products, Ltd.
P.O. Box 218
Dakota City, IA 50529
Phone: (515) 332-3087

Men's and women's vegan footwear (safety, athletic, hiking, dress), luggage, belts, baseball gloves, etc.

Mail Order Catalog
P.O. Box 180
Summertown, TN 38483
Phone: 1-800-695-2241

Extensive selection of vegan cookbooks. Also sells vegan food products, including tofu, TVP, nutritional yeast, and tempeh starter.

Micah Publications
255 Humphrey Street
Marblehead, MA 01945
Phone: (617) 631-7601

Books and materials about Judaism in relation to vegetarianism and animal rights.

Natural Lifestyle
16 Lookout Drive
Asheville, NC 28804-3330
Phone: 1-800-752-2775

Mail-order market for macrobiotic and organic foods and health-oriented "natural lifestyle" products, including cookware, personal-care products, housewares, clothing, and books.

The New Mountain Ark
799 Old Leicester Highway
Asheville, NC 28806
Phone: 1-800-643-8909

Carries a wide variety of macrobiotic foods, vegan foods, grains, beans, nuts, dried foods, and cooking equipment.

North American Vegetarian Society (NAVS)
P.O. Box 72
Dolgeville, NY 13329
Phone: (518) 568-7970

Offers a wide selection of books, videos, and products for vegan living.

Pangea
2381 Lewis Avenue
Rockville, MD 20851
Phone: (301) 652-3181

Carries a vast array of items including hard-to-find vegan food products (such as marshmallows), vegan shoes and accessories, books and personal-care products. Has both a retail store and a mail-order catalog.

Vegetarian Resource Group (VRG)
P.O. Box 1463
Baltimore, MD 21203
Phone: (410) 366-VEGE (8343)
Fax: (410) 366-8804

Vegan cookbooks, bumper stickers, postcards, pamphlets, etc.

Wild Wear
P.O. Box 31028
San Francisco, CA 94131
Phone: 1-800-428-6947
Fax: (415) 621-1435

T-shirts, sweatshirts, rubber stamps, magnets, pins, cards, and bumper stickers with animal-rights graphics and messages.

Vegan Products for Companion Animals

Evolution Diet
287 East Sixth Street, Suite 270
Saint Paul, MN 55101
Phone: (612) 228-0632 or (612) 228-0467

Makes vegan food for dogs, cats, and ferrets.

Harbingers of a New Age
717 East Missoula Avenue
Troy, MT 59935-9609
Orders: 1-800-884-6262
Phone: (406) 295-4944
Fax: (406) 295-7603

Supplies Vegepet products that provide essential nutrients for dogs and cats on a vegetarian or vegan diet. Also sells the book *Vegetarian Cats and Dogs,* by James A. Peden, which provides information and recipes that incorporate the Vegepet products.

Nature's Earth Products Inc.
510 Business Parkway
Royal Palm Beach, FL 33411
Phone: 1-800-749-PINE (7463)

Makes Feline Pine, a 100 percent pure, dust-free, odor-free, compostable, flushable, natural pine litter that is safe for your cat and the environment. Call to find the nearest retailer who carries it in your area.

Wow-Bow Distributors
13 B Lucon Drive
Deer Park, NY 11729
Phone: (516) 254-6064
Orders: 1-800-326-0230 (outside NY only)

Makes suitable supplements to fulfill a vegan dog's or cat's diet. Vegetarian and vegan biscuits, foods, and treats for companion animals and all farm animals, including rabbits and horses. Will custom create vegan products for specific animals' needs.

Wysong Corporation
1880 North Eastman Road
Midland, MI 48642-7779
Phone: (517) 631-0009
Fax: (517) 631-8801
Orders: 1-800-748-0188

Makes wet and dry vegan dog and cat foods.

Publications

Ahimsa
American Vegan Society (AVS)
56 Dinshah Lane
P.O. Box H
Malaga, NJ 08328
Phone: (609) 694-2887
Fax: (609) 694-2288

Free subscription to quarterly magazine with membership in American Vegan Society. Covers all issues related to vegan living.

The Animals' Agenda
1301 South Baylis Street
Suite 325
P.O. Box 25881
Baltimore, MD 21224
Phone: (410) 675-4566
Fax: (410) 675-0066
Subscriptions: 1-800-426-6884

Bimonthly magazine covering the full range of animal-rights issues and cruelty-free living.

Bunny Hugger's Gazette
P.O. Box 601
Temple, TX 76503
Fax: (254) 593-0116

Bimonthly newspaper covering animal protection issues, legislative campaigns, and events.

Good Medicine
Physicians Committee for Responsible Medicine (PCRM)
P.O. Box 6322
Washington, DC 20015
Phone: (202) 686-2210

This quarterly publication features news and articles on vegan nutrition, health, and animal research, as well as vegan recipes.

The McDougall Newsletter
P.O. Box 14039
Santa Rosa, CA 95402
Phone: 1-800-570-1654 or (707) 576-1654

A bimonthly nutrition newsletter focusing on very low-fat vegan eating with emphasis on health.

Natural Health
17 Station Street
Brookline, MA 02146
Subscriptions:
P.O. Box 7440
Red Oak, IA 51591
Phone: 1-800-526-8440

Bimonthly magazine with an emphasis on macrobiotics, alternative health care, and natural living. Not vegan, but has many vegan recipes and most articles are written with an appreciation of vegan views.

Vegetarian Journal
Vegetarian Resource Group (VRG)
P.O. Box 1463
Baltimore, MD 21203
Phone: (410) 366-VEGE (8343)

Free subscription to bimonthly magazine with membership to Vegetarian Resource Group. Covers issues related to vegetarian and vegan living. Recipes are strictly vegan.

Vegetarian Nutrition and Health Letter
Loma Linda University
1707 Nichol Hall, School of Public Health
Loma Linda, CA 92350
Phone: 1-888-558-8703 or (909) 478-8621

Eight-page nutrition newsletter written by Virginia Messina, M.P.H., R.D., and Mark Messina, Ph.D. Published ten times a year.

Vegetarian Times
P.O. Box 570
Oak Park, IL 60303
Phone: (708) 848-8100
Subscriptions: 1-800-435-9610

Monthly magazine featuring vegetarian recipes and articles related to vegetarianism.

Vegetarian Voice
North American Vegetarian Society (NAVS)
P.O. Box 72
Dolgeville, NY 13329
Phone: (518) 568-7970

Free subscription to quarterly magazine with membership in NAVS. Articles cover all aspects of vegan living. All recipes are strictly vegan.

Veggie Life
Box 440
Mount Morris, IL 61054-7660
Phone: 1-800-345-2785

Bimonthly magazine for "growing green, cooking lean, and feeling good." Vegetarian recipes and related articles.

RECOMMENDED READING

This is a very short list of recommended books related to vegan living, vegan philosophy, peace, and animal rights. There are many, many excellent books on these topics, so this compilation is by no means all inclusive—it's merely a jumping-off point.

Achor, Amy Blount. *Animal Rights: A Beginner's Guide.* Yellow Springs, Ohio: WriteWare, Inc., 1996.

Adams, Carol J. *The Sexual Politics of Meat: A Feminist-Vegetarian Critical Theory.* New York: Continuum Publishing Group, 1991.

American Vegan Society. *Here's Harmlessness.* Malaga, N.J.: American Vegan Society, 1993.

Arluke, Arnold, and Clinton R. Sanders. *Regarding Animals.* Philadelphia: Temple University Press, 1996.

Baker, Ron. *The American Hunting Myth.* Vantage Press, 1985.

Butler, C. T. Lawrence, and Keith McHenry. *Food Not Bombs: How to Feed the Hungry and Build Community.* Philadelphia: New Society Publishers, 1992.

Davis, Karen. *Prisoned Chickens, Poisoned Eggs: An Inside Look at the Modern Poultry Industry.* Summertown, Tenn.: Book Publishing Company, 1996.

Eisnitz, Gail A. *Slaughterhouse: The Shocking Story of Greed, Neglect, and Inhumane Treatment inside the U.S. Meat Industry.* Buffalo, N.Y.: Prometheus Books, 1997.

Fox, Michael W. *Super Pigs and Wondercorn: The Brave New World of Biotechnology and How It May Affect Us All.* New York: Lyons and Burford, 1992.

Francione, Gary L. *Animals, Property, and the Law.* Philadelphia: Temple University Press, 1995.

———. *Rain Without Thunder: The Ideology of the Animal Rights Movement.* Philadelphia: Temple University Press, 1996.

———, and Anna E. Charlton. *Vivisection and Dissection in the Classroom: A Guide to Conscientious Objection.* Jenkintown, Pa.: American Anti-Vivisection Society, 1992. (Available through American Anti-Vivisection Society.)

Free, Ann Cottrell. *No Room, Save in the Heart: Poetry and Prose on Reverence for Life—Animals, Nature & Humankind.* Washington, D.C.: Flying Fox Press, 1987. (Available through Flying Fox Press, 4204 Forty-fifth Street, NW, Washington, DC 20016.)

Hanh, Thich Nhat. *Peace Is Every Step: The Path of Mindfulness in Everyday Life.* New York: Bantam Books, 1991.

———. *Being Peace.* Berkeley, Calif.: Parallax Press, 1996.

Kowalski, Gary. *The Souls of Animals.* Walpole, N.H.: Stillpoint Publishing, 1991.

Lyman, Howard F. *Mad Cowboy: Plain Truth from the Cattle Rancher Who Won't Eat Meat.* New York: Scribner, 1998.

Marcus, Erik. *Vegan: The New Ethics of Eating.* Ithaca, N.Y.: McBooks Press, 1997.

Mason, Jim. *An Unnatural Order: Uncovering the Roots of Our Domination of Nature and Each Other.* New York: Simon and Schuster, 1993.

Mason, Jim, and Peter Singer. *Animal Factories.* New York: Crown Publishers, Inc. 1990.

Masson, Jeffrey Moussaieff, and Susan McCarthy. *When Elephants Weep: The Emotional Lives of Animals.* New York: Delacorte Press, 1995.

Nearing, Helen. *Loving and Leaving the Good Life.* Post Mills, Vt.: Chelsea Green Publishing, 1992.

Orwell, George. *Animal Farm.* Fiftieth Anniversary Edition. Estate of Sonia Brownell Orwell, 1995.

Peace Pilgrim: Her Life and Work in Her Own Words, compiled by some of her friends. Ocean Tree Books, 1992. (Available through Friends of Peace Pilgrim, 43480 Cedar Avenue, Hemet, CA 92544 or American Vegan Society.)

Quinn, Daniel. *Ishmael.* New York: Bantam Books, 1992.

Regan, Tom. *The Case for Animal Rights.* Berkeley, Calif.: University of California Press, 1983.

Regan, Tom, and Peter Singer, eds. *Animal Rights and Human Obligations.* Englewood Cliffs, N.J.: Prentice-Hall, 1989.

Roads, Michael J. *Talking with Nature.* Tiburon, Calif.: H.J. Kramer, Inc., 1987.

Rollin, Bernard E. *Animal Rights and Human Morality.* Prometheus Books, 1992.

Singer, Peter. *Animal Liberation.* New York: Avon Books, 1990.

Spiegel, Marjorie. *The Dreaded Comparison: Human and Animal Slavery.* Mirror Books, 1996. (Available through the Institute for the Development of Earth Awareness.)

Stull, Gordon D., Michael J. Broadway, and David Griffith, eds. *Any Way You Cut It: Meat Processing and Small-Town America.* University Press of Kansas, 1995.

Townend, Christine. *Pulling the Wool: A New Look at the Australian Wool Industry.* Hale and Iremonger, 1985. (Available through the American Vegan Society.)

BIBLIOGRAPHY

CHAPTER 3—The Way the West Was Weaned

Bath, Donald, et al. *Dairy Cattle: Principles, Practices, Problems, Profits.* Philadelphia: Lea and Febiger, 1985.

Bleifuss, Joel. "How Now Mad Cow?" *In These Times* 18, no. 5 (24 January 1994): 12–13.

Burke, B. P., and D. A. Funk. "Relationship of Linear Type Traits and Herd Life under Different Management Systems." *Journal of Dairy Science* 76, no. 9 (1993): 2773–2782.

Coghlan, Andy. "Arguing Till the Cows Come Home: European and American Regulators Lifted the Ban on the Sale of BST Treated Cow's Milk, but New Research Brings More Doubts." *New Scientist* 44, no. 1949 (29 October 1994): 14(2).

Dellorto, V., G. Savonini, and D. Cattaneo. "Effects of Recombinant Bovine Somatotropin (rBST) on Productive and Physiological Parameters Related to Dairy Cow Welfare." *Livestock Production Science* 36, no. 1 (1 July 1993): 71.

Firat, M. Z. "An Investigation into the Effects of Clinical Mastitis on Milk Yield in Dairy Cows." *Livestock Production Science* 36, no. 4 (1 November 1993): 311.

"Marathon Cow Sets World Record." *Associated Press,* 20 September 1996.

Milk Production, Report 5200, USDA National Agriculture Statistics, 1997. (This study was based on the average milk production per cow in twenty-two states in December 1996.)

Mohr, Paula. "More Milk Per Cow: Management and Genetics Boost Holstein Production Averages above 30,000 Pounds." *Farm Journal,* January 1996.

Sacks, Oliver. *An Anthropologist on Mars.* New York: Knopf Publishers, 1995.

Schwarz, A. "The Politics of Formula-Fed Veal Calf Production." *Journal of the American Veterinary Medical Association* 196, no. 10 (1990): 1578–86.

Strandberg, E. "Breeding for Longevity in Dairy Cows." *Progress in Dairy Science.* Edited by C. J. C. Phillips. Oxon, U.K.: CAB International, 1996.

Stull, C. L., and S. P. McDonough. "Multidisciplinary Approach to Evaluating Welfare of Veal Calves in Commercial Facilities." *Journal of Animal Science* 72 (1994): 2522.

Taylor, Robert E. *Scientific Farm Animal Production: An Introduction to Animal Science.* New York: Macmillan, 1991.

U.S. Department of Agriculture. *Agricultural Statistics.* 1986–1995.

U.S. Department of Agriculture. *Economic Opportunities for Dairy Cow Culling Management Options.* Animal and Plant Health Inspection Service (May 1996).

U.S. Department of Agriculture. *1996 Dairy Health and Health Management.* National Animal Health Monitoring System. APHIS Veterinary Services (November 1996).

U.S. Department of Agriculture. "1996 Dairy Health and Health Management Part 3." *National Animal Health Monitoring System* (1996).

U.S. Department of Agriculture. "1996 Dairy Management Practices." *National Animal Health Monitoring System* (1996).

U.S. Department of Agriculture. *Reference of 1996 Dairy Management Practices.* Animal and Plant Health Inspection Service. Fort Collins: Centers for Epidemiology and Animal Health (1996).

U.S. Department of Agriculture. *Qualitative Risk Assessment of BSE in the United States.* Animal and Plant Health Inspection Service. Fort Collins: Centers for Epidemiology and Animal Health (1991).

Walker, K. D., et al. "Comparison of Bovine Spongiform Encephalopathy Risk Factors in the United States and Great Britain." *Journal of the American Veterinary Medical Association* 199 (1991): 1554–61.

Webster, John. *Understanding the Dairy Cow.* Cambridge, Mass.: Blackwell Scientific, 1993.

Willeberg, P. "Bovine Somatotropin and Clinical Mastitis: Epidemiological Assessment of the Welfare Risk." *Livestock Production Science* 36, no. 1 (1 July 1993): 55.

———. "An International Perspective on Bovine Somatotropin and Clinical Mastitis." *Journal of the American Veterinary Medical Association* 205, no. 4 (1994): 538–41.

Wilson, Lowell L., Stanley E. Curtis, and Carolyn L. Stull. "Special Practices Produce Special-Fed Veal." *Hoard's Dairyman,* 10 August 1991.

CHAPTER 4—Which Came First?

Attia, Y. A., W. H. Burke, and K. A. Yamani. "Response of Breeder Hens to Forced Molting by Hormonal and Dietary Manipulations." *Poultry Science* 73, no. 2 (February 1994).

Damerow, Gail. *Chicken Health Handbook.* Williamstown, Maine: Storey Communications, 1994.

Davis, Karen. *Prisoned Chickens, Poisoned Eggs: An Inside Look at the Modern Poultry Industry.* Summertown, Tenn.: Book Publishing Co., 1996.

Elliott, Ian. "McDonald's Libel Suit Continues in London." *Feedstuffs*, 24 September 1995.

Fraser, David. *Food Animal Well Being 1993 Conference Proceedings and Deliberations*, "Assessing Animal Well Being: Common Sense, Uncommon Science." U.S. Department of Agriculture and Perdue University Office of Agricultural Research Papers. West Lafayette, Ind., 1993.

Gray, Carol V., Ph.D. "Poultry Pointers." *Lancaster Farming*, Lancaster, Penn., 18 July 1992.

Gregory, N. G., and L. J. Wilkins. "Broken Bones in Domestic Fowl: Handling and Processing Damage in End-of-Lay Battery Hens." *British Poultry Science* 30, no. 3 (September 1989).

Gussow, Joan Dye. "Ecology and Vegetarian Considerations: Does Environmental Responsibility Demand the Elimination of Livestock?" *American Journal of Clinical Nutrition* 59, no. 5 (1994): 5.

Knowles, T. G. "Handling and Transport of Spent Hens." *World's Poultry Science Journal* 50, no. 1 (March 1994).

Mitchell, M. A., and P. J. Kettlewell. "Road Transportation of Broiler Chickens: Induction of Physiological Stress." *World's Poultry Science Journal* 50, no. 1 (March 1994).

Mulhausen, J. R., et al. "Aspergillus and Other Human Respiratory Disease Agents in Turkey Confinement Houses." *American Industrial Hygiene Association Journal* 48 (1987): 894–99.

North, Mack O. *Commercial Chicken Production Manager*. Westport, Conn.: Avi Publishing, 1984.

Rollins, Bernard. *Farm Animal Welfare*. Iowa State University Press, 1995.

Taylor, Allison A., and J. Frank Hurnik. "The Effect of Long-Term Housing in an Aviary and Battery Cages on the Physical Condition of Laying Hens: Body Weight, Feather Condition, Claw Length, Food Lesions, and Tibia Strength." *Poultry Science* 73, no. 2 (February 1994).

"The Egg Industry of California and the USA in the 1990s: A Survey of Systems." *World's Poultry Science Journal* 49, no. 1 (March 1993).

U.S. Congress. Office of Technology Assessment. *Impacts of Antibiotic Resistant Bacteria*. OTA-H-629. Washington, D.C.: Government Printing Office, September 1995.

U.S. Department of Agriculture. *Chickens and Eggs*. Washington, D.C.: NASS, July 21, 1998

Whyte, R. T. "Aerial Pollutants and the Health of Poultry Farmers." *World's Poultry Science Journal* 49, no. 2 (July 1993).

Zayan, Rene, and Ian J. H. Duncan. *Cognitive Aspects of Social Behavior in the Domestic Fowl*. New York: Elsevier Science, 1987.

CHAPTER 5—Invisible Oppression

American Heart Association. *1998 Heart and Stroke Statistical Update.* Dallas: 1997.

Anding, Jenna D., et al. "Blood Lipids, Cardiovascular Fitness, Obesity, and Blood Pressure: The Presence of Potential Coronary Heart Disease Risk Factors in Adolescents." *Journal of the American Dietetic Association* 96, no. 3 (1996): 238–42.

Cooper, Marc. "The Heartland's Raw Deal: How Meatpacking Is Creating a New Immigration Underclass." *The Nation* 264, no. 4 (3 February 1997): 11.

"David Fights Goliath in Northern Missouri." *Farm Aid Update.* Champaign, Ill., 1995.

Gardner, Gary. "Preserving Agricultural Resources." *State of the World 1996.* Edited by Linda Starke. New York: W. W. Norton, 1996.

General Accounting Office. "School Lunch Program: Role and Impacts of Private Food Service Companies." August 1996.

Harris, William, M.D. *The Scientific Basis of Vegetarianism.* Honolulu: Hawaii Health Publishers, 1996.

Hedges, Stephen J., Dana Hawkins, and Penny Loeb. "Illegal in Iowa/The New Jungle." *U.S. News & World Report,* 23 September 1996, 34–45.

Horowitz, Tony. "9 to Nowhere." *The Wall Street Journal,* 1 December 1994, A1.

Meadows, Robin. "Livestock Legacy." *Environmental Health Perspectives* 103, no. 12 (December 1995).

Norvell, Candyce. "Why Is Everyone Griping about School Lunches: Poor Nutrition in School Food Programs." *Current Health 2* 21, no. 5. (January 1995): 27.

"Organizing the Poultry Industry." *UFCW Action.* United Food and Commercial Workers Union, November/December 1995.

Raymond, Jennifer, M.S. "Helping School Lunches Make the Grade." *Vegetarian Voice* 22, no. 3 (Fall 1997).

Robbins, John. *May All Be Fed: Diet for a New World.* New York: Avon Publishing, 1992.

Sachs, Aaron. "Upholding Human Rights and Environmental Justice." *State of the World 1996.* Edited by Linda Starke. New York: W. W. Norton, 1996.

Starke, Linda, ed. *Vital Signs 1996: Trends That Shape Our Future.* Worldwatch Institute. New York: W. W. Norton, 1996.

Stull, Donald D., Michael J. Broadway, and David Griffith. *Any Way You Cut It: Meat Processing and Small-Town America.* Lawrence: University of Kansas Press, 1995.

CHAPTER 6—Environment in Crisis

Abdalla, Charles W., Les E. Lanyon, and Milton C. Hallberg. "America: What We Know about Historical Trends in Firm Location Decisions and Regional Shifts: Policy Issues for an Industrializing Animal Sector." *Journal of Agricultural Economics* 77, no. 5 (December 1995): 1229.

Ausubel, Kenny. *Seeds of Change: The Living Treasure.* San Francisco: Harper, 1994.

Barnet, Richard J., and John Cavanagh. *Global Dreams: Imperial Corporations and the New World Order.* New York: Simon & Schuster, 1994.

Brown, Lester. *State of the World.* New York: W. W. Norton, 1976.

Cantrell, Patty, Rhonda Perry, and Paul Sturtz. "Hog Wars: The Environment and Factory Farms in the Corporate Grab for Control of the Hog Industry and How Citizens Are Fighting Back." Columbia, Missouri Rural Crisis Center, Mo.: 1997.

Cockburn, Alexander. "Dead Meat." *The Nation* 262, no. 16 (22 April 1996): 9.

Comly, H. H. "Cyanosis in Infants Caused by Nitrates in Well Water. *Journal of the American Medical Association* 257 (1987): 2788–92.

Danaher, Kevin. "Introduction: Corporate Power and the Quality of Life." In *Corporations Are Gonna Get Your Mama: Globalization and the Downsizing of the American Dream*. Monroe, Maine: Common Courage Press, 1996.

Di Silvestro, Roger. "Your Tax Dollars Are Feeding Cattle and Destroying Habitat." *National Wildlife* 34, no. 1 (December/January 1995): 58.

Durning, Alan. *How Much Is Enough: The Consumer Society and the Future of the Earth*. New York: W. W. Norton, 1992.

———. "Fat of the Land." *World Watch* 4, no. 3 (May–June 1991): 11–17.

———, and Holly B. Brough. "Taking Stock: Animal Farming and the Environment." World Watch paper no. 103. Washington, D.C.: Worldwatch Institute, 1991.

"Environmental Indicators for Agriculture." Paris, France: Organisation for Economic Co-Operation and Development, 1997.

Environmental Working Group. "Pouring It On: Nitrate Contamination of Drinking Water." Washington, D.C., February 1996.

Farm Aid. "David Fights Goliath in Northern Missouri." Champaign, Ill., spring 1995.

Gillespie, James R. *Modern Livestock and Poultry Production*. San Francisco: Delmar Publishers, 1997.

Glover, Mike. "Study Shows Environmental Risks of Animal Waste." Associated Press, 28 December 1997.

Goering, Peter, Helena Norber-Hodge, and John Page. *From the Ground Up: Rethinking Industrial Agriculture*. Berkeley, Calif.: International Society for Ecology and Culture, 1993.

Harris, William, M.D. *The Scientific Basis of Vegetarianism*. Honolulu: Hawaii Health Publishers, 1996.

Howlett, Debbie. "Lakes of Animal Waste Pose Environmental Risk." *USA Today*. 30 December 1997.

Hunter, Beatrice Trum. "What Is Fed to Our Food Animals?" *Consumer's Research Magazine* 79, no. 12 (December 1996): 13.

Jacobs, Lynn. *Waste of the West: Public Lands Ranching*. Tucson, Ariz.: Lynn Jacobs, 1991.

Jensen, Carl. *Censored: The News That Didn't Make the News and Why*. New York: Four Walls Eight Windows, 1995.

Kross, B. C., et al. "The Nitrate Contamination of Private Well Water in Iowa." *American Journal of Public Health* 83 (1993): 270–72.

Lehman, Karen. *Dinner at the Global Cafe: It's Tough to Swallow*. Minneapolis: Institute for Agricultural and Trade Policy, February 1995.

Lynch, Eamon. "What Price Pigs? A Massive Spill Points Out the Problems with Factory Farms." *Audubon* 97, no. 5 (September/October 1995): 14.

Mason, Jim. "The Beast Within." *E: The Environmental Magazine*. November/December 1995.

Meadows, Robin. "Livestock Legacy." *Environmental Health Perspectives.* 103, no. 12 (December 1995).

Morse, Deanne. "Impact of Environmental Regulations on Cattle Production." *Journal of Animal Science* 74 (1996): 3103–11.

"Murphy's Laws: (1) Hogs Rule (2) You Pay." *Sierra* 81, no. 3 (May–June 1996): 29.

Myers, Norman. *Gaia: An Atlas of Planet Management.* Revised and updated edition. New York: Anchor Books, 1993.

Pimentel, David. "Environmental and Economic Benefits of Sustainable Agriculture." *Neue Partnerschaften in der Marktwirtschaft oder Okologische Selbstzerstorung* (Vienna): Bundesministerium fur Land und Forstwirtschaft, special issue of *Forderungsdienst* (1992): 95–109.

———. "Environmental and Economic Costs of Pesticide Use: An Assessment Based on Currently Available U.S. Data, Although Incomplete, Tallies $8 Billion in Annual Costs." *Bioscience* 42, no. 10 (November 1992): 750–60.

———. "Impact of Population Growth on Food Supplies and Environment." *Bioscience,* presented at AAAS Annual Meeting, Baltimore, Md., February 9, 1996.

———. "Livestock Production: Energy Inputs and the Environment." In *Canadian Society of Animal Science.* S.L. Scott and Xin Zhao, eds. Proceedings, 47th Annual Meeting, Montreal, Quebec, 24–26 July 1997, 16–26.

———, and Mario Giampietro. "Food, Land, Population and the U.S. Economy." Carrying Capacity Network, Washington, D.C., 21 November 1994.

———, and Henry W. Kindall. "Constraints on the Expansion of the Global Food Supply." *Ambio* 23, no. 3 (May 1994).

———, et al. "Conserving biological diversity in agricultural/forestry system." *Bioscience* 42 (1994): 354–62, as printed in Pimentel and Giampietro.

———, et al. "Water Resources: Agriculture, the Environment and Society." *Bioscience* (in press) as printed in "Impact of Population Growth on Food Supplies and Environment," presented at AAAS Annual Meeting, Baltimore, Md. February 9, 1996.

Rifkin, Jeremy. *Beyond Beef: The Rise and Fall of the Cattle Culture.* New York: Dutton, 1992.

Rogers, Adam. "Taking Action: An Environmental Guide for You and Your Community." U.N. Environment Programme in association with the U.N. Non-Governmental Liaison Service, 1996.

Satchell, Michael. "Hog Heaven and Hell: Pig Farming Has Gone High Tech and That's Creating New Pollution Woes." *U.S. News & World Report,* 22 January 1996.

Segelken, Roger. "U.S. Could Feed 800 Million People with Grain that Livestock Eat, Cornell Ecologist Advises Animal Scientists," press release. Montreal, 7 August 1997.

Shiva, Vandana. *Biopiracy: The Plunder of Nature and Knowledge.* Boston: South End Press, 1997.

Spiegel, Marjorie. *The Dreaded Comparison: Human and Animal Slavery.* New York: Mirror Books, 1996.

Stauber, John, and Sheldon Rampton. *Toxic Sludge Is Good for You: Lies, Damn Lies and the Public Relations Industry.* Monroe, Maine: Common Courage Press, 1995.

Stith, Pat, and Joby Boss Warrick. "Hog: North Carolina's Pork Revolution." *The News & Observer,* 19–26 February 1995.

Todd, Betsy. "The Effects of Diet on the Environment." *Imprint* (April/May 1994).

U.S. Department of Agriculture. Natural Resources Conservation Service. Ecological Sciences Division. *Animal Manure Management,* December 1995. NRCS/RCA Issue Brief 7.

Wuerthner, George. "Alien Invasion: Exotic Plant and Animal Species Are One of the Gravest Threats to the Native Flora and Fauna of the National Parks." *National Parks* 70, nos. 11–12 (November/December 1996): 32–34.

———. "The Price Is Wrong." *Sierra.* (September/October 1990): 40–41.

CHAPTER 7—Shooting the Myths

Archery Loss in Texas. Texas Parks and Wildlife Department, 1987.

Decker, Daniel J., Jody W. Enck, and Tommy L. Brown. "The Future of Hunting: Will We Pass on the Heritage?" *Second Annual Governor's Symposium on North America's Hunting Heritage Proceedings;* North American Hunter, North American Hunting Club, and Wildlife Forever, Minnetonka, Minn., undated.

"Deer Hunting Retrieval Rates." *Michigan Pittman-Robertson Report,* 1984.

Fund for Animals. *Hunting Fact Sheet No. 1: An Overview of Killing for Sport.* Compiled by the Fund for Animals with data from the U.S. Fish and Wildlife Service and state wildlife agencies. New York: Fund for Animals, 1997.

Maryland Department of Natural Resources. Forest, Park, and Wildlife Service. "Maryland Wild Turkey Report." Lansing, Md.: Maryland Department of Natural Resources, 1989.

Michigan Department of Natural Resources. Wildlife Division. "Management Direction for Southern Michigan Wildlife: A Strategic Plan for Managing Southern Michigan's Wildlife Resources." Lansing, Md.: Michigan Department of Natural Resources, 1991.

Missouri Department of Conservation. 1987. *Survey of Archery Hunters.*

———. 1989. "Species Management Plan for the Ring-Necked Pheasant in Missouri," Wildlife Division.

New South Wales, Australia. 1988. *New South Wales Animal Welfare Advisory Council on Duck and Quail Shooting.* Report. (Although this report specifically covers the state of New South Wales, Australia, duck hunting with shotguns is practiced similarly in Australia as in North America.)

South, Rob. "The Economics of Hunting." In *Second Annual Governor's Symposium on North America's Hunting Heritage Proceedings.* Minnetonka, Minn.: North American Hunter, North American Hunting Club, and Wildlife Forever, undated.

U.S. Fish and Wildlife Service. "Number of Paid Hunting License Holders, License Sales, and Cost to Hunters: Fiscal Year 1995." Report. Washington, D.C.: U.S. Fish and Wildlife Service, undated.

CHAPTER 8—Animals and Entertainment

Chavez, Cesar. Letter to Eric Mills dated 26 December 1990. Printed with permission.

Finley, Bill. "Sadly No Way to Stop Deaths." *New York Daily News,* 10 June 1993.

Fund for Animals. *Marine Mammal Fact Sheet No. 1: Cetaceans in Captivity; Dolphins: An Overview.* New York: Fund for Animals, undated.

———. *Marine Mammal Fact Sheet No. 2: Cetaceans in Captivity; Orcas: An Overview.* New York: Fund for Animals, undated.

Greyhound Protection League. "Know the Facts About Greyhound Racing and Animal Exploitation." Woodside, Calif.: March 1997.

Hanauer, Gary. "The Killing Tanks." *Penthouse* (October 1989).

Humane Society of the U.S. (HSUS). "Help Keep Whales and Dolphins Free." Washington, D.C.: undated.

———. "Horse Slaughter Fact Sheet." Washington, D.C.: 1994.

———, and the American Humane Association (AHA). Joint Policy Statement, 5 May 1982.

Karasik, Gary. "You Can Bet Their Life on It." *Miami Herald Tropic,* 21 October 1990.

Knowles, Joseph. "Saving Grace: The Life of a Retired Athlete." *Chicago Sports Profiles,* June 1994.

Lambert, Florence. "No Place for Elephants." *The Washington Post,* 1 April 1995.

Lamm, Shelby Stockton. "Circus Practices Are Cruel to Animals." *The Journal Gazette,* 22 October 1995.

McClintock, Jack. "Run or Die." *Life* 14 (June/July 1991).

McKenna, Virginia, Will Travers, and Jonathan Wray, eds. *Beyond the Bars: The Zoo Dilemma.* Rochester, Vt.: Thorsons, 1987.

Maggitti, Phil. "Uneasy Riders." *Town & Country* 147, no. 5155 (April 1993).

Michelmore, Peter. "Hidden Shame of an American Sport." *Reader's Digest* 141, no. 844 (August 1992): 103.

Pacelle, Wayne. "Horse Racing: What's Around the Bend?" *The Animals' Agenda* 8, no. 5 (June 1988): 16.

Performing Animal Welfare Society (PAWS). *The Circus: A New Perspective.* Galt, Calif.: Performing Animal Welfare Society, 1996.

Reitman, Judith. "The Greatest Shame on Earth?" *Fairfield County Advocate,* 11 September 1989.

Rose, Naomi A. Letter to the editor, *National Geographic Traveler* 12 (3 February 1995).

———. "Marine Mammals in Captivity." *The Animals' Agenda* 16, no. 3 (July/August 1996).

Schoon, Nickolas. "Animal Groups Say Zoos Fool the Public." *The Independent,* 6 July 1994.

"Troubled Marine Park to Close." *Associated Press,* 3 July 1994.

Van Valkenburg, Scott, and Rebecca Taksel. "Free Willy . . . Free Them All." *The Animals' Agenda,* January/February 1994.

William, Jonathan. *The Rose-Tinted Menagerie.* London: Heretic Books Ltd., 1990.

CHAPTER 9—Science: Fact, Fiction, or Fantasy

Allen, Scott. "Group Says Mexican Cats Sold for U.S. Dissection Die Cruelly by Drowning." *Boston Globe,* 24 March 1994.

Altman, Lawrence. "Doctors Treating AIDS Patient Turn to Baboon Marrow Cells." *The New York Times,* 15 December 1995.

Associated Press. "Doctors Call Use of Baboon Livers 'Bad Science.'" 1 February 1993.

———. "Cats Stolen, Drowned for Dissection." 24 March 1997.

Bailar, J., and H. Gornik. "Cancer Undefeated." *New England Journal of Medicine* 336, no. 22 (29 May 1997).

———, and E. M. Smith. "Progress Against Cancer." *New England Journal of Medicine* 314 (1986): 1226–32.

Colburn, Don. "Organ Donations Hinge on Survivors' Consent." *The Washington Post,* 4 August, 1995, Health Section.

Doris, Margaret. "The Animal Within: The Risks and Ethics of Trans-Species Transplants." *New York Perspectives,* 16 October 1992.

Drayer, Mary Ellen, ed. *The Animal Dealers: Evidence of Abuse of Animals in the Commercial Trade, 1952-1997.* Washington, D.C.: Animal Welfare Institute. 1997.

Ethical Science Education Committee. 1995. *The Frog Fact Sheet.* Boston: Ethical Science Edcation Committee.

———. 1995. *The Turtle Fact Sheet.* Boston: Ethical Science Education Committee. Sources cited: Barbara Bonner, D. Eng, and O. Feingold. "Bacteriology in Wild and Warehoused Red-eared Slider Turtles, Trachemys scripta elegans" (13th International Herpetological Symposium on Captive Propagation and Husbandry); M. Uricheck, and Barbara Bonner, eds., unpublished data, 1989; Barbara Bonner, "Veterinary Care of Moribund Red-eared Slider Turtles, Trachemys scripta elegans," notes from talk given at Wildlife Disease Association Annual Meeting, El Paso, Texas, 1992.

Fox, Michael W. *Super Pigs and Wondercorn: The Brave New World of Biotechnology and How It May Affect Us All.* New York: Lyons and Burford, 1992.

Michaels, Marian, and Richard Simmons. "Xenotransplant-Associated Zoonoses." *Transplantation* 57 (1994): 1–7.

More, D., and C. L. Ralph. "A Test of Effectiveness of Courseware in a College Biology Class." *Journal of Educational Technology Systems* 21 (1992): 79–84.

Phillips, Mary T. "Savages, Drunks, and Lab Animals: The Researcher's Perception of Pain." *Society and Animals* 1, no. 1 (1994).

Reitman, Judith. *Stolen for Profit.* New York: Kensington Publishing, 1992.

Rowan, Andrew, Franklin Loew, and Joan Weer. "The Animal Research Controversy: Protest, Process, and Public Policy—an Analysis of Strategic Issues." Boston: Center for Animals and Public Policy, 1995.

Russell, W. M., and R. L. Burch. *The Principles of Humane Experimental Technique.* London: Methuen and Co. Science, 1959.

Sabin, Albert. Transcripts from testimony to the House Committee on Veterans Affairs, 1984.

Samsel, R.W., et al. "Cardiovascular Physiology Teaching: Computer Simulations vs. Animal Demonstrations." *Advances in Physiology Education* 11 (1994): S36–S46.

Secretary of Agriculture, *Animal Welfare Enforcement.* Report to the President of the Senate and the Speaker of the House of Representatives. 1996.

Sharpe, Robert. *The Cruel Deception: The Use of Animals in Medical Research.* Northamptonshire, England: Thorsons Publishing Group, 1988.

———. *Science on Trial.* Sheffield, England: Awareness Publishing, 1994.

Smith, Dean. "International Trade in Pets for Dissection." *The AV Magazine* 102, no. 5 (May 1994): 8–10.

Steele, David J. R., and Hugh Auchincloss. "The Applications of Xenotransplantation in Humans—Reasons for Delay." *ILAR Journal* 37, no. 1 (1995): 13–15.

Stephens, M. *Advances in Animal Welfare Science* (1986/87): 19–31.

National Association of Biology Teachers. *The Responsible Use of Animals in Biology Classrooms.* Policy statement. Reston, Va.: National Association of Biology Teachers, 1989.

Thompson, Dick. "Giving Up on the Mice." *Time,* 17 September, 1990.

CHAPTER 10—The Compassionate Consumer

Australia Bureau of Statistics. Catalogue 7721.0 (1991–92).

Clifton, Merritt. "The Myth of the Good Shepherd." *The Animals' Agenda,* May 1990.

Dinshah, Jay. "Why Vegans Don't Use Honey." *Ahimsa,* July/September 1991.

D'Silva, Joyce. "Horrors on the Sheep Farm." *Agscene* 84 (July 1986): 2–3.

Ensminger, M. E. *Beef Cattle Science.* Danville, Ill.: Interstate Printers and Publishers, 1997.

Gang, Elliot L. "The Buzz About Honey." *The Animals' Agenda,* November/December 1997.

Macauley, Dave. "From Craft to Commodity: Leather and the Leather Industry." *The Animals' Agenda,* September/October 1988.

Moran, Victoria. "Going Non-leather." *The Animals' Agenda,* March 1992.

National Cattlemen's Beef Association. *Cattle and Beef Industry Statistics.* National Cattlemen's Beef Association (March 1996).

Pyevich, Caroline. "Busy Bees." *Vegetarian Journal,* November/December 1996.

Reilly, Lee. "Whether Leather?" *Vegetarian Times,* October 1994.

"Rising Deathtoll in Live Sheep Export." *Animals Today,* November 1994–January 1995.

Ryder, Michael L. "The Evolution of the Fleece." *Scientific American,* January 1987.

Senate Select Committee on Animal Welfare. "Sheep Husbandry." Canberra, Australia: Government Publishing Service, 1989.

Short, Charles E., and Alan Van Poznak. *Pain in Animals.* New York: Churchill Livingstone, 1992.

U.S. Department of Agriculture. *1994 Sheep Death Loss Due to Predators and Health-Related Causes.* Veterinary Services Information Sheet, 1996.

Vegan Society. "Wool Report." London: The Vegan Society, 1997.

Wolfson, Elissa. "Toward Sustainable Shoes." *E: The Environmental Magazine,* November/December 1990.

INDEX